Physical Therapy of the Hip

CLINICS IN PHYSICAL THERAPY

EDITORIAL BOARD

Otto D. Payton, Ph.D., **Chairman**
Louis R. Amundsen, Ph.D.
Suzann K. Campbell, Ph.D.
Jules M. Rothstein, Ph.D.

Physical Therapy of the Hip

Edited by
John L. Echternach, Ed.D., P.T.

Professor and Chairman
School of Community Health Professions
and Physical Therapy
Director
Program in Physical Therapy
College of Health Sciences
Old Dominion University
Norfolk, Virginia

CHURCHILL LIVINGSTONE
New York, Edinburgh, London, Melbourne

Library of Congress Cataloging-in-Publication Data

Physical therapy of the hip / edited by John L. Echternach.
     p.   cm. — (Clinics in physical therapy)
    Includes bibliographical references.
    Includes index.
    ISBN 0-443-08650-8
    1. Physical therapy. 2. Hip—Diseases—Patients—Rehabilitation.
I. Echternach, John L. II Series.
    [DNLM: 1. Hip—physiopathology. 2. Physical Therapy. W1CL831CN
v. 21 / WE 855 P578]
RM700.P474 1990
617.5′81—dc20
DNLM/DLC
for Library of Congress   90-2060
                                                                  CIP

Distributed in the United Kingdom by Churchill Livingstone, Robert Stevenson
House, 1–3 Baxter's Place, Leith Walk, Edinburgh EH1 3AF, and by associated
companies, branches, and representatives throughout the world.

Accurate indications, adverse reactions, and dosage schedules for drugs are provided
in this book, but it is possible that they may change. The reader is urged to review the
package information data of the manufacturers of the medications mentioned.

The Publishers have made every effort to trace the copyright holders for borrowed
material. If they have inadvertently overlooked any, they will be pleased to make the
necessary arrangements at the first opportunity.

Acquisitions Editor: *Kim Loretucci*
Copy Editor: *Elizabeth Bowman*
Production Designer: *Gloria Brown*
Production Supervisor: *Jeanine Furino*

Printed in the United States of America

First published in 1990

Contributors

Thomas E. Croley, Ph.D.
Associate Professor of Anatomy, School of Physical Therapy, Texas
Woman's University, Dallas, Texas

John L. Echternach, Ed.D., P.T.
Professor and Chairman, School of Community Health Professions and
Physical Therapy, and Director, Program in Physical Therapy, College of
Health Sciences, Old Dominion University, Norfolk, Virginia

John L. Echternach, Jr., M.S., P.T.
Physical Therapist, Professional Therapies of Roanoke, Roanoke, Virginia

Louis R. Jordan, M.D.
Associate Professor, Department of Orthopedic Surgery, Eastern Virginia
Medical School of the Medical College of Hampton Roads, Norfolk, Virginia

Deborah King-Echternach, B.S., P.T.
Pediatric Physical Therapist, Rehabilitative Services of Roanoke, Roanoke,
Virginia

Susan D. Lambert, P.T., S.C.S., A.T.C.
Sports Physical Therapist, Physical Therapy Specialty Center; Athletic
Trainer, Tidewater Sharks Minor Professional Football Team; Instructor,
Sports Physical Therapy Curriculum, Old Dominion University, Norfolk,
Virginia

George C. Maihafer, M.S., P.T.
Associate Professor, School of Community Health Professions and Physical
Therapy, College of Health Sciences, Old Dominion University, Norfolk,
Virginia

Carol A. Oatis, Ph.D., P.T.
Co-Director, Philadelphia Institute for Physical Therapy, Philadelphia; Adjunct Assistant Professor, Department of Physical Therapy, Beaver College, Glenside, Pennsylvania

Curtis V. Spear, Jr., M.D.
Associate Professor and Chairman, Department of Orthopedic Surgery, Eastern Virginia Medical School of the Medical College of Hampton Roads, Norfolk, Virginia

Evangeline Yoder, M.S., P.T.
Associate Professor, School of Community Health Professions and Physical Therapy, College of Health Sciences, Old Dominion University, Norfolk, Virginia

Preface

The role of the hip in ambulation and in posture is of central importance to physical therapy. However, in looking at current continuing education offerings, and the field's literature, there seems to be much more clinical concern for physical therapy management of low back, shoulder, and knee problems than for the management of hip problems.

One of the purposes of this text is to focus attention on the hip and provide physical therapists with a source for the clinical management of patients with hip problems. A blend of basic sciences and clinical material was felt to be desirable to achieve this; therefore, this book covers the basic sciences of anatomy of the hip in Chapter 1, evaluation of the hip in Chapter 2, and biomechanical considerations and the role of the hip in posture and gait in Chapters 3 and 9. Since it is important to understand the pathologic processes and the medical and surgical management of the hip, these topics are covered in Chapters 4 and 5. Chapters 6 and 7 provide the framework for managing both surgical and non-surgical hip problems. Because, in our society, increasing sports activity is a phenomenon that cannot be overlooked, we have included a chapter on sports injuries to the hip (Chapter 8). The final two chapters in the book discuss hip problems in two special clinical populations —- children and adolescents and the elderly —- in which management may sometimes significantly differ from management of the general adult population.

I would like to thank the contributing authors to this text for taking the time out of their busy lives to share their insights into hip problems with the readers. I would also like to thank especially Deborah Miller for the illustrations for several of the chapters in the text as well as Alex Leidholdt for his photography. Illustrations and photographs add immeasurably to the printed material, and we are indeed indebted.

In addition I would like to acknowledge two others for their contributions in a very indirect way to this text. Early in my career I was fortunate enough to work with a physical therapist named Joseph Hoog. He was the most astute physical therapy clinician that I had encountered in my early career. His example created for me an indelible impression of the importance of clinical observation and analysis as the foundation for physical therapy practice. Secondly, I would like to acknowledge the contributions of my wife, Jeanne, for being a patient soundingboard and listener as well as one who offers wise counsel, particularly when things are not going the way that I would like them to. Her advice on this and many other things has always been important.

John L. Echternach, Ed.D., P.T

Contents

1 | Anatomy of the Hip

Thomas E. Croley

The hip joint is a ball-and-socket (spheroidal diarthroses) joint between the head of the femur and the acetabulum of the hip bone. The joint must possess great strength for supporting the entire weight of the body plus movement forces and at the same time allow a wide range of movements accomplished during the body's locomotion. The hip joint serves for weight transmission since it connects the lower limb to the trunk. As an illustration, just think of the many forces exerted on this single joint in a simple catapult maneuver by a gymnast.

OSTEOLOGY OF THE HIP JOINT

Os Coxae

Anatomic Relationships

The os coxae (hip bone) is the lateral contribution of the bony pelvis. In childhood it consists of three individual bones. These three bones fuse, and this fusion takes place for all three bones primarily within the acetabulum, the concavity constructed for the reception of the head of the femur (Fig. 1-1). The ilium, which forms the superior portion of the os coxae, also forms the superior two-fifths of the acetabulum. The pubis forms the anterior portion of the os coxae, as well as the anteromedial one-fifth of the acetabulum.

Fusion of Ilium, Ischium, and Pelvis

The three fusion lines can be seen within the acetabulum (Fig. 1-1).
The fusion of the ischial ramus with the inferior ramus of pubis creates a protuberance that can be seen projecting into the obturator foramen.

1

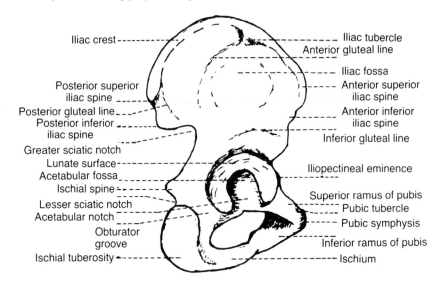

Fig. 1-1.   The os coxae—lateral view.

The fusion of the body of the ilium with the body of the pubis creates the ridge known as the iliopubic (iliopectineal) eminence (Figs. 1-1 and 1-2).

General Characteristics of Os Coxae

Obturator Foramen.   The obturator foramen is an oval opening created by the fusion of the pubic and ischial bones. The bodies of each bone fuse to form the inferior boundary of this foramen.

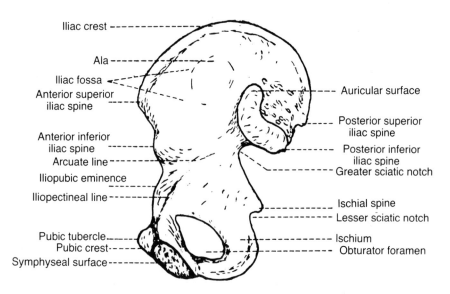

Fig. 1-2.   The os coxae—medial view.

An obturator groove can be found within the anterosuperior portion of the foramen that serves for the passage of the obturator nerve and vessels out of the pelvis. During life, this foramen is enclosed by an obturator membrane except for the above-mentioned area of passage for the obturator nerves and vessels.

Acetabulum. The acetabulum is the concavity constructed for the reception of the head of the femur. It is formed by the fusion of the ilium, ischium, and pubis. From birth until puberty, these bones are separated by a Y-shaped area of articular, hyaline cartilage. This cartilage is replaced by bone at 15 to 17 years of age. The acetabulum is constructed with a central depression, the fossa, surrounded by an articular portion, the lunate surface. This articular surface surrounds the fossa peripherally except in the inferior region where it leaves a gap, the acetabular notch (Fig. 1-1).

Linea Terminalis. The os coxae contribute to the linea terminalis, which is a circumferential plane that creates a lateral border for the opening between the greater and lesser pelvis known as the pelvic brim. The posterior portion of the linea terminalis, known as the arcuate line, is a ridge on the pelvic surface of the ilium coursing from the sacrum to the iliopubic eminence (Fig. 1-2). This ridge separates the body from the ala of the ilium. The anterior portion of the linea terminalis, known as the iliopectineal line, courses from the iliopubic eminence anteriorly to the superior crest of the symphysis pubis.

Specific Characteristics of Individual Bones

Ilium. The curved superior margin of the ilium is known as the iliac crest. This crest is easily palpable on the inferior portion of the flank or side of the body. The most superior extent of the crest occurs at the level of the fourth lumbar vertebra. This crest serves as a marker to determine this important landmark. Just anterior to this highest point of the crest, there is a thickening that is roughened on its superior surface known as the tubercle of the crest. This tubercle is 5 to 6 cm posterosuperior from the anterior superior iliac spine and serves as the attachment site for the iliotibial tract (band).

The iliac crest extends anteriorly to form the anterior superior iliac spine by abruptly ending, with the anterior margin of the bone continuing inferiorly. This spine is easily palpated and in thin individuals can be seen protruding beneath the skin.

The iliac crest extends posteriorly to abruptly end as the posterior superior iliac spine. This spine is difficult to palpate but can be located in some individuals from the skin and underlying fasciae attached to the spine, which create a surface dimple superficial to this attachment.

The anterior and posterior margins curve inward below these anterior and posterior superior iliac spines and then curve outward again to form anterior and posterior inferior iliac spines, respectively.

The external surface of the iliac bone presents three lines on the ala or flattened surface. An inferior gluteal line extends posteriorly from the notch between the two anterior spines and is slightly curved inferiorly. An anterior gluteal line extends from just posterior to the anterior superior iliac spine and courses posteroinferiorly in a curved manner to end in front of the greater sciatic notch. A posterior gluteal line extends from the midpoint of the posterior one half of the iliac crest and courses inferiorly to end at the greater sciatic notch, as do the other gluteal lines. These lines are ridges of excess bone created by the tension resulting from the margins of various gluteal muscles.

The greater sciatic notch is an exaggerated concavity within the posterior margin of the ilium just below the posterior inferior iliac spine. It serves for the passage of the large sciatic nerve as it exits the pelvis.

The internal surface of the iliac bone has a depression, the iliac fossa, that serves for the origin of the iliacus muscle.

At the most posterior region of the internal surface of the iliac bone, there is an ear-shaped surface, hence the name auricular surface, for articulating the sacrum (Fig. 1-2).

Between the auricular surface and the posterior end of the crest is an area that is quite roughened and contains depressions. This area, the tuberosity, serves for attachment of ligaments, such as the interosseous ligaments for supporting the sacroiliac joint.

A ridge, the arcuate line, extends obliquely below the iliac fossa and forms the posterior end of the linea terminalis. The body of the iliac bone is located below this line and contributes to the formation of the acetabulum.

Ischium. The ischium is the L-shaped bone of the os coxae having a very prominent, roughened tuberosity on its posterior portion for ligament attachment and serving for origin of the hamstring muscles (Fig. 1-1). Superior to the tuberosity is a thickened portion of the bone. This is the body, and it forms two-fifths of the acetabulum. Anteromedially from the tuberosity projects the flattened portion of the bone, the ramus, which fuses with the inferior ramus of the pubis. The posterior margin of the body has a projection that protrudes posteromedially, the spine, which serves for attachment of the sacrospinous ligament and superior gemellus muscle. Inferior to the spine, the posterior margin indents into a concavity to form the lesser sciatic notch. The area on the posterolateral side of the body and between the tuberosity and the acetabulum is deeply grooved for the passage of the tendon of the obturator externus muscle.

Pubis. The pubis can be divided into a body and a superior and an inferior ramus (Figs. 1-1 and 1-2). The flattened body of one pubic bone joins that of the opposing pubic bone to form the symphysis pubis joint of the bony pelvis. The superior margin of the body has a prominent projection, the tubercle, and a ridge extending medially from this tubercle, which is the crest of the pubic bone. Extending superolaterally from the tubercle and crest along the superior ramus is a prominent ridge, the pecten pubis, which as it passes more toward the iliac bone becomes known as the iliopectineal line. This iliopectineal line terminates into the iliopubic eminence at the commencement of the arcuate line. This flattened inferior ramus of the pubis extends inferolaterally from the body to contribute to the formation of the inferior margin of the obturator foramen. The junction with the ramus of the ischium produces a protuberance where the inferior ramus of the pubis terminates.

Femur

This strong bone of the thigh articulates with the os coxae in a unique manner. The width of the pelvis varies from individual to individual. The pelvis is normally wider in women than in men; therefore, the femur must angle more obliquely in women to articulate at the knee joint along the line of gravity for the inferior extremity. It is thought that this causes some of the knee problems seen in clinics.

The proximal end of the femur consists of a head, a neck, and a greater and lesser trochanter. A ridge of bone extends between the trochanters on both the anterior and posterior sides, that on the posterior being markedly larger (Fig. 1-3). The trochanters are located on the proximal (upper) end of the shaft of the bone, which receives the neck at an oblique angle. This angle is approximately 125° with the longitudinal axis of the body in the adult, but varies considerably throughout life and between sexes.

The head of the femur is smooth except for a depression, the fovea capitis, which serves for the attachment of the ligamentation capitis femoris.

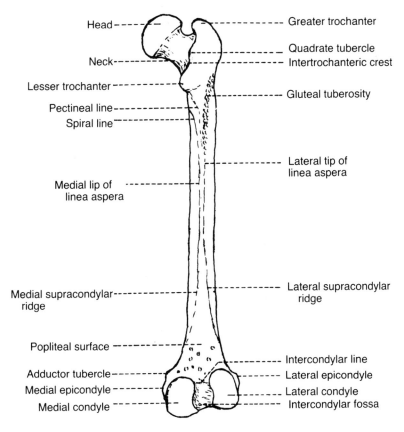

Fig. 1-3.   The femur—posterior view.

The smooth surface of the head abruptly ends in a ridge encircling the head, which rapidly gets smaller in diameter to form the neck. The neck has numerous nutrient foramina for branches of the femoral circumflex arteries to give this region adequate blood supply.

The greater trochanter extends above the junction of the neck and has a depression on its medial side, the trochanteric fossa. The superior surface of the greater trochanter has two impressions for musclar attachment. One is antero-medial and serves for the attachment of the obturator internus and gemelli muscles. The other, which is posterolateral, serves for attachment of the piri-formis muscle. The medial surface of the greater trochanter has an impression in the superior portion of the trochanteric fossa for the attachment of the obturator externus muscle. The lateral surface of the greater trochanter has a semicircular impression that serves for the attachment of the gluteus medius muscle. The anterior surface of the greater trochanter has a flattened impression for the attachment of the gluteus minimus muscle.

The lesser trochanter, located posteromedially, has an impression for the attachment of the iliopsoas muscle tendon. On the posterior surface and extend-ing between the greater and lesser trochanters there is a prominent ridge, the intertrochanteric crest. On this crest, a prominence, the quadrate tubercle, serves as the attachment for the quadratus femoris muscle. On the anterior surface, extending between the trochanters, is a roughened line serving pri-marily for ligament attachment, the intertrochanteric line (Fig. 1-4). An incon-spicuous raised area is found near the cranial end of this line, the femoral tubercle, which serves primarily for the attachment of the ischiofemoral lig-ament.

The inferior extent of the intertrochanteric line can be followed around to the medial and then to the posterior surface as it becomes the spiral line, which ends by coursing inferolaterally until meeting the linea aspera. A roughened ridge, the gluteal tuberosity, extends superolaterally from the cranial end of the linea aspera, and serves for the attachment of the gluteus maximus muscle. Between these two cranial projections of the linea apsera is a much less conspic-uous ridge, the pectineal line, which extends upward to the lesser trochanter and serves as the site of attachment for the pectineus muscle. These cranial projections converge inferiorly into a raised, prominent crest as the cranial end of the linea aspera, which extends inferiorly and occupies the middle one-third of the posterior surface. The linea aspera has a medial and a lateral lip and extends inferiorly until these lips diverge to form the medial and lateral supra-condylar ridges. The linea aspera serves as the attachment site for many of the thigh muscles. The medial supracondylar ridge ends distally as the raised, adductor tubercle, which receives the tendon of the adductor magnus muscle. The posterior smooth surface between the supracondylar ridges is the popliteal surface.

The distal end of the femur is expanded to form the medial and lateral condyles. These condyles are separated posteriorly by a deep intercondylar fossa demarcated from the popliteal surface by a ridge, the intercondylar line. The condyles blend together on the anterior surface to form the patellar articular

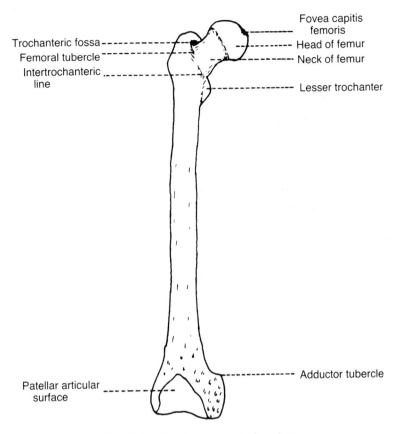

Trochanteric fossa

Femoral tubercle

Intertrochanteric line

Fovea capitis femoris

Head of femur

Neck of femur

Lesser trochanter

Adductor tubercle

Patellar articular surface

Fig. 1-4. The femur—anterior view.

surface. The articular surfaces of the condyles are unequal—that of the lateral condyle presents more articular surface with the patella, creating a larger surface on the patella.

Roughened raised areas above the femoral condyles create the medial and lateral epicondyles, which serve as the attachment sites for the medial and lateral collateral ligaments.

ARTHROLOGY AND LIGAMENTS OF THE HIP JOINT

Sacroiliac Articulation

Ventral Sacroiliac Ligaments

The ventral sacroiliac ligaments create a thin layer connecting the ventrolateral surface of the sacrum to the ventral margin of the auricular surface of the ilium. Coursing across the superoventral surface of this layer are the superior and inferior portions of the iliolumbar ligament.

Dorsal Sacroiliac Ligaments

The dorsal sacroiliac ligaments course from the posterior superior and posterior inferior iliac spines inferiorly and medially to attach to the tubercles of the lateral sacral crest (Fig. 1-5). The short dorsal sacroiliac ligaments attach to the first and second tubercles, whereas the long dorsal sacroiliac ligaments attach to the third and fourth tubercles of the lateral sacral crest.

Interosseous Ligaments

The interosseous ligaments course from the iliac tuberosity downward and medially across to the sacral tuberosity. They are very short, strong fibers that are deep to the dorsal sacroiliac ligaments. They give the sacroiliac joint much of its stability.

Sacroischial Articulation

Sacrotuberous Ligament

The sacrotuberous ligament begins as a broad base originating from the posterior inferior iliac spine across to the third and fourth tubercles of the lateral sacral crest and to the lateral surface of the sacrum. These fibers converge as they pass inferiorly and insert on the medial portion of the ischial tuberosity.

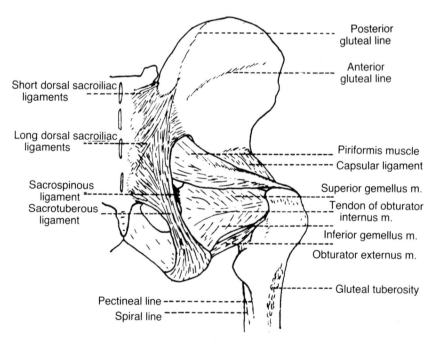

Fig. 1-5.   The posterior hip with associated muscles and ligaments.

This ligament, along with the sacrospinous ligament, encloses the greater and lesser sciatic notches, thus creating the sciatic foramina.

Sacrospinous Ligament

The sacrospinous ligament is ventral to the sacrotuberous ligament (Fig. 1-5). Its fibers are attached to the lateral margins of the sacrum and coccyx and course laterally and inferiorly in a convergence to attach to the spine of the ischium.

Sacrococcygeal Articulation

Ventral Sacrococcygeal Ligaments

The ventral sacrococcygeal ligaments consist of a scant amount of fibers that descend from the ventral surface of the apex of the sacrum down to the ventral surfaces of the coccygeal vertebrae. They blend with the descending anterior longitudinal ligament and periosteum of the vertebral column.

Dorsal Sacrococcygeal Ligaments

The dorsal sacrococcygeal ligaments consist of a layer of fibers that descend from the dorsal surface of the bodies of the sacral vertebrae within the sacral canal and hiatus down to the dorsal surfaces of the coccygeal vertebrae. They blend with the fibers of the posterior longitudinal ligament and periosteum of the vertebral column.

Lateral Sacrococcygeal Ligaments

The lateral sacrococcygeal ligaments consist of a few fibers that descend from the lateral surface of the sacrum down to connect with the transverse processes of the coccygeal vertebrae.

Interposed Fibrocartilage

The interposed fibrocartilage consists of a cartilaginous disc similar to that found in contiguous vertebrae above except for lacking a nucleus pulposus.

Interarticular Ligaments

The interarticular ligaments consist of two strands of fibers interconnecting the cornu of the sacrum with those of the first coccyx.

Pubic Symphysis

Superior Pubic Ligament

The superior pubic ligament consists of strands of fibers passing from the pubic crest on one side of the pubic joint. These fibers blend with the interpubic disk between the two pubic bones.

Arcuate Pubic Ligament

These fibers course from the inferior margin of the inferior ramus of the pubis across to connect to the inferior margin of the opposing pubic bone. In doing so, they form an arch along the bony pubic arch of the pelvis. These fibers blend with those of the interpubic disc.

Interpubic Disc

The interpubic disc is a layer of fibrocartilage intervening between the opposing articular surfaces of the two pubic bones. The fibrocartilage blends with a layer of hyaline cartilage next to the bony surfaces that is held on by many Sharpey's fibers embedded into the bony tissue.

Acetabular Joint and Associated Ligaments

Capsular Ligament

The capsular ligament surrounding the hip joint attaches anteriorly along the intertrochanteric line and posteriorly around the neck just superior to the intertrochanteric crest. The capsule is continuous around the joint with three major thickenings: the iliofemoral ligament and pubofemoral ligament anteriorly and the ischiofemoral ligament posteriorly.

Iliofemoral Ligament

The iliofemoral ligament is an anterior thickening of the capsule of the hip joint consisting of very strong fibers. These fibers pass from the anterior inferior iliac spine and diverge into two major bands that fan out to attach along the intertrochanteric line. This arrangement forms an inverted Y, thus the synonym, Y ligament of Bigelow.

Pubofemoral Ligament

The pubofemoral ligament is an anterior and medial thickening of the capsule of the hip joint. These fibers pass from the superior ramus of the pubis over the obturator foramen and pass laterally and inferiorly to insert along the intertrochanteric line of the femur deep to the fibers of the iliofemoral ligament.

Ischiofemoral Ligament

The posterior thickening of the capsule of the hip joint, the ischiofemoral ligament, consists of fibers that spiral around the neck of the femur to the anterior side, thus creating the anatomic screw-home mechanism for this joint. The fibers pass from the posterior ridge of the ischium dorsal to the acetabulum and spiral anteriorly around the neck of the femur to attach to the femoral tubercle at the summit of the intertrochanteric line. Therefore, when the thigh is extended, these spiraled fibers tighten. Conversely, when the thigh is flexed, these spiraled fibers loosen (uncoil), making the posterior capsule flexible and weakened.

Ligamentum Capitis Femoris

The lunate surface of the acetabulum is covered with a fibrocartilage layer called the acetabular labrum because it extends peripherally over the edge of the acetabulum. As this layer approaches the notch of the acetabulum, the tissue takes on more fibers, which extend across the notch to form the transverse ligament.

The transverse acetabular ligament serves as the origin for the ligamentum capitis femoris, a triangular ligament that will pass into the acetabular fossa to attach to the fovea of the head of the femur. It is inside this ligament that the branch of the obturator artery passes to enter and supply the head of the femur.

Innervation to Capsule and Ligaments of Acetabular (Hip) Joint

The anterior portion of the capsule receives nerve fibers from the femoral and obturator (posterior division) nerves. The posterior portion of the capsule receives nerve fibers from the nerve to the quadratus femoris muscle and superior gluteal nerve.

MYOLOGY OF THE HIP JOINT

Gluteus Maximus

The largest and thickest muscle within the gluteal region is the gluteus maximus muscle. Its fibers descend in an inferior and lateral direction. It arises from the iliac bone posterior to the posterior gluteal line and along the sacro-tuberous ligament and the dorsal sacroiliac ligaments. Fibers course from these sites downward to insert by way of a superficial and deep portion. The superficial insertion is into the iliotibial tract. The deep insertion is into the gluteal tuberosity of the femur. A large trochanteric bursa is found deep to this muscle as it passes over the greater femoral trochanter.

On the deep, inferior portion of the muscle can be found the inferior gluteal nerve as it passes into the red belly fibers for motor innervation. This muscle receives its blood supply by way of both the superior and the inferior gluteal arteries, as they pass above and below the underlying piriformis muscle to enter the gluteus maximus and other gluteal muscles. Based on these origins and insertions, this muscle is one of the strong extensors and lateral rotators of the hip joint.

Gluteus Medius

The fibers of the gluteus medius muscle, just deep to the gluteus maximus muscle, are more vertical than that muscle. Each of the two muscles is invested by its own deep investing fascia and separated by branches of the inferior and superior gluteal vessels.

The gluteus medius muscle arises from the external surface of the ilium between the posterior and anterior gluteal lines. The red belly fibers pass inferiorly to insert in a curved manner along the superior and lateral surfaces of the greater trochanter of the femur.

On the deep surface of the muscle is located the superior gluteal nerve and branches that supply motor innervation to the muscle. Accompanying these motor branches are superior and inferior gluteal vessels that also supply this muscle. This muscle is involved in abduction and pelvic support when only one foot is on the ground and the other is raised. This is the muscle most involved in the Trendelenburg test.

The Gluteus Minimus

The gluteus minimus is a rather thin muscle situated between the gluteus medius muscle and the external surface of the ilium. Its fibers course vertically downward, and it is separated from the overlying gluteus medius by branches of the superior gluteal nerve and the superior gluteal and inferior gluteal vessels.

The gluteus minimus muscle arises from the external surface of the ilium between the anterior and inferior gluteal lines. Its fibers pass inferiorly and slightly posteriorly to insert into a facet on the anterior surface of the greater trochanter of the femur.

The superficial surface of the gluteus minimus has numerous branches of the superior gluteal nerve entering it to supply it with motor innervation. On this surface as well are numerous branches of the superior and inferior gluteal vessels that also supply it. Owing to the direction that the fibers course to insert, this muscle functions as a medial rotator of the thigh, as well as abducting the thigh and maintaining the stability of the pelvis.

Piriformis

Owing to the particular arrangement of the structures within the gluteal region, the piriformis serves as a landmark for the region. The superior gluteal nerve and vessels course out above the piriformis muscle, while the inferior gluteal nerve and vessels course out below the muscle. The very large sciatic nerve courses out below the muscle along with the nerve to the obturator internus muscle, the nerve to the quadratus femoris muscle, and the pudendal nerve and internal pudendal vessels.

The piriformis muscle arises from the anterior surfaces of sacral vertebrae two, three, and four. The muscle along with the related structures above and below all pass out of the pelvis through the greater sciatic foramen. The red belly fibers converge into an obvious tendon that passes laterally to insert into the superior and medial border of the greater trochanter of the femur.

The pelvic surface of the muscle, just as it arises, has some of the sacral plexus of nerves coursing across it. The ventral primary rami of sacral nerves one and two extend branches into this surface for innervation to the muscle. The superior and inferior gluteal vessels supply the piriformis as they exit on either side of it.

Obturator Internus

The red belly fibers of the obturator internus muscle arises from the internal (pelvic) surface of the bony obturator foramen and membrane. These fibers converge into a tendon as the muscle exits the pelvis through the lesser sciatic foramen. The posterior view of the gluteal region shows the tendon coursing out of the gluteal region just below the spine of the ischium and passing laterally to insert on the medial surface of the greater trochanter of the femur. Just before this insertion, the gemelli muscles can be seen inserting into the tendon of the obturator internus muscle.

The arterial supply to the obturator internus and accompanying gemelli muscles is by way of branches off of the cruciate anastomosis. The cruciate anastomosis is made up of anastomotic connections between the inferior gluteal, medial femoral circumflex, lateral femoral circumflex, and first perforating arteries. The medial femoral circumflex artery sends branches up to interconnect with the inferior gluteal artery, and as this takes place over the obturator internus and gemelli muscles, branches pass into these muscles for their vascular supply. The nerve to the obturator internus muscle is a nerve that exits off the sacral plexus and passes into the superficial side of the muscle and the related superior gemellus for motor innervation to the two muscles.

Gemelli

The fibers of the superior gemellus arise from the ischial spine, while those of the inferior gemellus arise from the most superior portion of the ischial tuberosity. The red belly fibers of both muscles converge to insert on opposite sides of the tendon of the obturator internus muscle before its insertion.

The blood supply to both muscles and motor innervation to the superior gemellus have been discussed with the obturator internus muscle. The motor nerve to the inferior gemellus muscle is derived from the nerve to the quadratus femoris muscle off of the sacral plexus. The obturator internus and gemelli muscles assist in abduction of the thigh and lateral rotation of the thigh. They also help to stabilize the head of the femur within the acetabulum.

Quadratus Femoris

The quadratus femoris muscle is a short, rectangular muscle situated below the inferior gemellus muscle. Its fibers arise from the lateral border of the ischial tuberosity and pass laterally to insert into the quadrate tubercle on the intertrochanteric crest of the femur.

Characteristically, the medial femoral circumflex artery will course deep to the quadratus femoris muscle and exit above and below the muscle with branches. Therefore, the muscle receives its blood supply by way of this artery and receives motor innervation from a specialized nerve branch off of the sacral plexus. The quadratus femoris muscle is a strong lateral rotator of the thigh. Deep to this muscle lies the ischiofemoral portion of the capsule of the hip joint.

VASCULAR SUPPLY OF THE HIP JOINT

The anterior portion of the neck of the femur and the anterior portion of the capsule of the hip joint are supplied by the lateral femoral circumflex artery, in contrast to the posterior portion of the neck of the femoral and the posterior portion of the capsule, which are supplied by the medial femoral circumflex artery. These two arteries branch off the profunda femoris artery within the femoral triangle of the thigh. The head of the femur receives a branch from the obturator artery. The two femoral circumflex arteries anastomose around the femoral trochanters and contribute to the trochanteric and cruciate anastomoses. The superior portion of the capsule is supplied by the gluteal vessels that contribute to the anastomoses around the joint.

The arterial vessels described all have venal commitantes that are responsible for circulating the blood back to the femoral vein for venous return.

CUTANEOUS NERVE SUPPLY OVER THE HIP REGION

The posterior gluteal region receives cutaneous nerves from superior, lateral to inferior, and medial by way of the subcostal nerve, the iliohypogastric nerve, the dorsal primary rami of L1, L2, L3, and the dorsal primary rami of S1, S2, and S3, consecutively. These dorsal primary rami along with cutaneous branches off the posterior femoral cutaneous nerve are many times referred to as clunial nerves.

The anterior region of the hip has its cutaneous supply divided around the inguinal ligament. Superior to this ligament the region is innervated by the iliohypogastric nerve. Inferior to the ligament there are three cutaneous areas. The superior area is innervated by the subcostal nerve, the intermediate by the femoral branch of the genitofemoral nerve, and the inferior region by the iliolingual nerve (Fig. 1-6).

SUMMARY

From the study of the anatomy of the hip it is evident why it can perform its normal functions with the strength and stability that it maintains. This is clearly appreciated when a patient has to adjust initially to a new hip prosthesis. Yet,

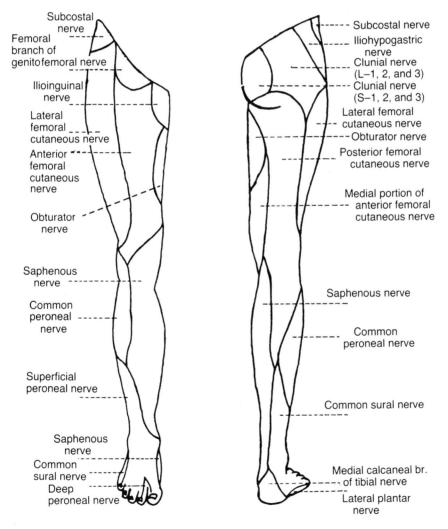

Fig. 1-6. Cutaneous innervation of the lower extremity.

when one studies the hip joint in several pelvises, the individual variability can also be appreciated. Remember, the human body and its parts must never be taken for granted, but must be appreciatively taken care of throughout life.

In the pages that follow, the complexities of the anatomy of the hip and the importance of this area in the clinical examination and management of problems of the region will become evident. This region offers challenges to the clinician because of the central importance of the hip in weightbearing, standing, and walking. An appreciation of the anatomy of this area is fundamental to all that follows in this text.

SUGGESTED READING

1. Hollinshead WH: Anatomy for Surgeons. Vol. 3. 2nd Ed. Harper & Row, New York, 1969
2. Hollinshead WH, Rosse C: Textbook of Anatomy. 4th Ed. p. 349. Harper & Row, New York, 1985
3. Moore KL: Clinically Oriented Anatomy. 2nd Ed. Williams & Wilkins, Baltimore, 1984
4. Palastanga N, Field D, Soames R: Anatomy and Human Movement, Structure and Function. Ch. 5. Heinemann Medical Books, Portsmouth, NH, 1989
5. Sobotta J: Atlas of Human Anatomy. Vol. 1. Figge FE (ed). Hafner, New York, 1974

2 | Evaluation of the Hip

John L. Echternach

This chapter discusses the evaluation (examination) of the hip region. At one time when discussing the physical therapist's evaluation of the hip or any other area it was assumed that the patient was referred by another health care practitioner. Since that assumption is no longer necessarily true, it becomes even more important that physical therapists possess well developed skills in evaluation (examination). Obviously examination of the patient is only one part of the scheme for the patient's care, but it is usually the starting place for anything else that a physical therapist will do with a patient with a hip problem. Since this is so, this chapter has two primary purposes: to state the components of an acceptable hip region examination (see Appendix 2-1) and to provide information that will help the physical therapist develop proficiency in performing an examination of the hip region. Physical therapists can then use this information to fit into the overall plan for care of a patient.

The profession of physical therapy has created some confusion about the use of the terms evaluation and examination. Originally physical therapists used the word *evaluation* primarily to avoid any indication that what the physical therapist did had diagnostic implications; thus, use of the word evaluation has become well entrenched among physical therapists. However, the word has caused difficulties for some time because evaluation implies a judgment in which we are attributing value to the information derived. A more exact definition of what this chapter covers would be the use of the word *examination*. Examination implies the gathering of facts and information concerning a topic without making a value judgment about the information gathered.

An examination of an area is essentially the use of a series of measurements and tests of that area. As we have become a more mature profession, our literature has discussed objective and subjective tests.[1-3] Many of the tests used by clinicians are highly subjective but are often not questioned, even though the subjectivity of the measurement seems to be well understood. It may be worth repeating that subjectivity refers to the amount of interpretation of any measurement that the examiner brings to the test situation, even though what is being measured may appear to be objective.[1] From time to time as we go through the examination process we will discuss this issue in relationship to particular tests being performed. The ultimate role of the examination of any region is to provide the examiner with information that will play a major role in planning appropriate treatment for the patient. The information derived from this examination will be used in setting goals and determining future progress of the patient towards those goals.[4] Patients, whenever possible, should be involved in this goal-setting process because, after all, it is the patient's goals that are important, not the therapist's goals.[4]

THE EXAMINATION PROCESS

As we go through this examination process, please refer to Appendix 2-1, which outlines the process and shows the type of information being gathered in each section. The examination process begins with defining the patient's problem. The first contact with the patient in this examination process usually involves gathering information about the patient's present complaint. The problem-oriented method helps in documenting the examination process. Once the problem has been clarified, then information about the problem becomes important. This includes such things as history, previous treatment, onset of the problem, and any information that the patient has available to share with the examiner from previous contacts with health professionals concerning this problem. In an institutional environment, this will often include a chart which the therapist would review, that includes a great deal of data about the patient. No source of information available to the therapist should be overlooked before beginning the physical portion of the examination. Obviously in a clinical environment there are constraints about how much time can be spent in this data gathering before examining the patient, and it is hoped that the physical therapist will use common sense in alloting time and effort to gathering this data.

Subjective Information

Subjective information will be gathered from the patient. This information will include information about the patient's chief complaint (problem), particularly information about pain. When information is gathered about pain, the more specific the information is, the more helpful it is to the therapist in determining how this pain relates to the patient's overall problem. So it is important to have the patient describe the type and location of pain, what activities may increase the pain, what activities relieve the pain, whether the pain is constant or cyclical, and whether the patient perceives the pain problem as increasing or lessening. Since the hip joint is a weightbearing joint it is very important to gather information concerning the role of weightbearing in pain activities, particularly whether the patient has pain at rest as well as during weightbearing, or whether specific activities (e.g., stair climbing and walking) are the cause of increased pain.

Objective Information

In conducting the examination itself, several methods or strategies have been proposed.[5-10] Most of these schemes are adequate, and it is incumbent upon the examiner to become familiar enough with a particular method of examination so that the process is a comfortable and familiar one. When discussing or describing an examination strategy, it is difficult to describe the process in ways that are always understandable in terms of the "flow" of the examination. For instance, if you look at the method proposed by Hoppenfeld,[5] the major headings are inspection, bony palpation, soft tissue palpation, range of motion (ROM), neurologic examination, special tests, and examination of related areas. Such a scheme is very comprehensive and would cover all of the important information as you filled in the areas between major headings to complete the examination. One of the difficulties in explaining such a scheme is that the patient will be standing for some of the activities, sitting for some of the activities, and in a supine or prone position for some of the activities; therefore the flow of the examination depends on the experience of the examiner in knowing not only the scheme, but also the positions that the patient should be in when the examination is being carried out. If one were to slavishly follow this scheme from top to bottom, the patient and the examiner would be wasting a great deal of time in changing positions for each of the new phases of the examination. So as we discuss the examination process, it should be kept in mind that we are describing the kinds of information that need to be gathered, not necessarily the order in which they will be gathered or the patient's position when the information is being gathered.

Another difficulty in learning an examination scheme is that a complete examination would cover nearly all possibilities for detecting information in the area, whereas when carrying out the examination in the clinical environment sometimes a point can be reached in which the clinician decides the information gained makes further investigation in that particular area unnecessary. The process of examination is best taught in the clinical environment by an experienced clinician in a close relationship with the learner. At this point it becomes important for the clinician teacher to be able to verbalize the thought processes that go with the examination process, or explain how decisions are reached that determine what is next in the examination and the meaningfulness of the information gathered from the patient.

Observation and Inspection

The first step in the physical examination process is observation and inspection, which begins with the first contact with the patient. The examiner observes the patient's arrival to determine the following:

1. What assistive device was needed for arrival (e.g., a wheelchair, crutches, canes)
2. Does the patient appear to be in pain or comfortable
3. Does the patient have any obvious asymmetries in muscle contours, any obvious leg length discrepancies, or any obvious foot position abnormalities (e.g., one foot markedly inwardly or outwardly rotated)

While observing the patient, also note whether the pelvis is level. An easy way to detect this is to have the patient stand, place your hands on top of the iliac crests, and observe whether they are level. Also inspect the buttock and thigh regions for muscle atrophy or asymmetry, for obvious discolorations of the skin, and for swollen areas around the pelvis and thigh.

Palpation

The next step in conducting the physical examination would be in palpating for areas of tenderness, nodules, masses, spasm of large muscles, etc., in the region. Hoppenfeld[5] suggests an approach to palpation that is organized by region, separating bony palpation from soft tissue palpation. Organization of the examination in this way is very helpful to the examiner, since it improves the possibility of doing the procedures in an organized and complete fashion. Even though Hoppenfeld separates bony palpation from soft tissue palpation, the two can be done concurrently in the sense that when you are examining the anterior aspect bony palpation, you would also be doing the soft tissue palpation for this area. The examination proceeds as follows.

Anterior Aspect Bony Palpation. The therapist examines the anterior superior iliac spine, the iliac crest, the iliac tubercle, the greater trochanter, and the pubic tubercles. These are all available for palpation when the examiner is anterior to the patient. This examination is often done with patients in the standing position supporting themselves against the treatment table. Because the iliac crest is part of this palpation process, this is one easy point at which pelvic obliquity could be determined. Each of these suggested areas is an important bony landmark. The greater trochanters are easily palpated in the superior portion, and should be level and easily found. The anterior iliac spine is an important landmark for muscle attachments and also assists in finding the iliac crest and the iliac tubercle. The iliac tubercle is the widest portion of the pelvis.

Posterior Aspect for Bony Palpation. The patient is usually put in a side-lying position so that the following bony prominences can be palpated: the posterior superior iliac spines, the greater trochanter again, the ischial tuberosity, and the sacroiliac joint (Fig. 2-1). The sacroiliac joint in this position cannot be palpated directly because of the overlying ilium as well as several ligaments; however, certain bony landmarks here are important. From the crest of the ilium an imaginary line can be drawn that would place the examiner between the L4 nd L5 spinous processes. The same is true for the sacroiliac joint in that a line

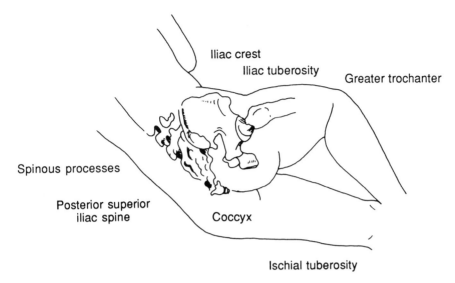

Iliac crest

Iliac tuberosity

Greater trochanter

Spinous processes

Posterior superior
iliac spine

Coccyx

Ischial tuberosity

Fig. 2-1. The important bony landmarks of the pelvis and hip with the patient in the side-lying position.

drawn from the posterior superior iliac spine to the midline crosses S2 and the center of the sacroiliac joint.[5] Since the hip joint itself is deep to muscles and other structures, it cannot be palpated directly; therefore, other sources of information must be used to gain information directly about the hip joint.

Soft Tissue Palpation. In the soft tissue palpation, certain basic structures need to be examined. In the anterior aspect it is important to palpate for the femoral triangle and for the femoral artery pulse. The vein and the nerve passing through the femoral triangle ordinarily are not able to be palpated directly. However, the relationship between the palpable femoral artery and the nerve and vein are important; the vein is the most medial structure and the nerve the most lateral structure in the femoral triangle. For examining the femoral triangle, the patient is supine and, if it is possible for the patient to do this, has the heel of the leg examined resting upon the opposite knee (Fig. 2-2). This puts the patient in a position of flexion-abduction and external rotation. Also palpable in this anterior position is the inguinal ligament, which extends from the medial pubic tubercle laterally to the anterior superior iliac spine.

Muscles in the area of the femoral triangle are the sartorius and the adductor longus (Fig. 2-2). The sartorius muscle forms the lateral border of the femoral triangle and can be palpated at its origin. In the position described earlier, or the patient with his knee flexed and his heel on his opposite knee with the hip in the adducted position, the proximal tendon of the adductor longus is prominent and can be easily palpated. Dancers, cheerleaders, and others who perform strenuous activity requiring abduction at the hip often will have strained this muscle, and it may be tender to palpation.

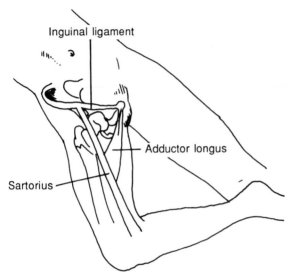

Inguinal ligament

Adductor longus

Sartorius

Fig. 2-2. The relationships of various structures around the femoral triangle, important during the palpation portion of the examination.

Going from the anterior aspect to the lateral aspect, palpation of the greater trochanter is important because of the possibility of trochanteric bursitis. Often this area is tender. The bursa itself cannot be palpated unless it is tender or inflamed. Also, the gluteus medius muscle inserts into the upper portion of the trochanter and can be palpated laterally.

Posteriorly one of the most important of the soft tissue areas to palpate is the sciatic nerve. This can be located midway between the greater trochanter and the ischial tuberosity when the patient is in the side-lying position described earlier for the bony palpation portion of the posterior portion of the region (Fig. 2-1). There are a number of causes of tenderness of the sciatic nerve, including piriformis muscle spasm and direct trauma to the nerve itself. Also in this position a bursa overlying the ischial tuberosity can be palpated. Usually the patient's history would lead to examination of this area.

A group of techniques are used for examining whether bursa are inflamed in the hip region. The first is the previously mentioned bursa around the greater trochanter, or subtrochanteric bursa. A method for testing this is to carry the patient's leg into hyper-adduction (across the midline), ask the patient to abduct the hip while you resist the motion. As the hip abductors contract they compress the bursa, causing discomfort in the area of the greater trochanter. The same principle can be applied to the psoas bursa, which lies beneath the iliopsoas muscle; as the iliopsoas contracts over this inflamed bursa, it can cause pain in the inguinal region. A patient is placed in the position of abduction, and flexion and pain is noted on resisted motion. Hoppenfeld[5] has described a bursa beneath the gluteus maximus. If it becomes inflamed it does not cause joint pain, but pain in the lateral aspect of the hip, particularly when the hip is resisted in going into extension.

Most of the muscles that are superficial and cross the hip region can be palpated. An approach to palpation of muscles is to divide them into groups by function: the flexor group, the adductor group, the abductor group, and the extensor group. Since manual muscle testing of the hip joint is also part of the examination, it is possible to do the muscle palpation portion of the examination at the same time that the examiner does the manual muscle testing.

Range of Motion

Both active and passive ROM should be determined. Testing should be performed using a goniometer for documentation. The examiner should record which portion of the ROM is pain free and which portion causes the patient to feel pain.

Initially, passive ROM can be performed primarily to see what portion of the ROM might be causing difficulties, particularly in pain or in decreased motion. After this evaluative portion of ROM testing, specific ROM testing should be done and recorded.

Active ROM in hip flexion is 0° to 120°. Passive ROM into hip flexion often is available to 135°. Hip flexion should be examined in the supine position. Hip abduction is from 0 to 45 to 50°, and should also be examined in the supine position. Hip adduction can be carried out from 20° to 30° crossing the midline with the one leg crossing over the top of the other. Hip extension is usually 0° to 20° and should be performed, when possible, with the patient in the prone position. Hip rotation should be performed with the patient sitting with internal rotation of 0° to 35° and external rotation of normally 0° to 45°.

Information on "normal" hip ROM must be viewed with some skepticism since very little age-related information on hip ROM is available. I have cited the most commonly used figures for ROM of the hip.

In addition to routine ROM testing, several special tests that have ROM implications can be performed around the hip joint. The first of these is the Thomas test for hip flexion contracture (Fig. 2-3). In the Thomas test the uninvolved hip is flexed as far as possible and stabilized while the involved hip is expected to be in the zero, or neutral, position. Measurements are taken of the amount of flexion that the involved hip demonstrates when the uninvolved hip is fully flexed. Bringing the patient's uninvolved hip into the flexed position flattens the pelvis and stabilizes the hip joint. This makes the flexion of the involved hip visible and clearly demonstrates the origin of the loss of extension to the hip. Patients with flexion contractures can not extend the involved leg without arching their lumbar spine, for which the examiner should palpate when performing this test (Fig. 2-3).

Another test that can be performed that has ROM implications is the Ober test. In this test the patient is instructed to lie in the side-lying position with the uninvolved leg flexed towards the chest so that the top leg should adduct to the point where it touches the examining table. If a patient has tightness of the iliotibial band, then the involved leg will not lower to the treatment table.

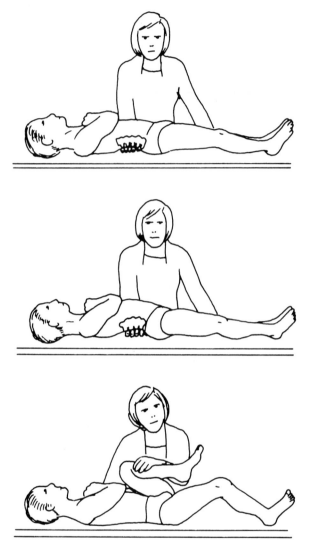

Fig. 2-3. The Thomas test for hip flexion contracture. The top illustration shows the spine in the normal position, the middle illustration shows that a patient with tight hip flexors will have an increased lumbar lordosis with the legs extended, the bottom illustration shows how by flexing the uninvolved leg as far as possible the pelvis is stabilized showing the amount of hip flexion contracture in the involved leg.

Cyriax[10] describes the "sign of the buttocks." In patients with posterior hip pain he performs first a straight leg raising examination. If the patient has pain in the buttocks with straight leg raising, this would indicate a lumbar nerve root problem. If the patient has pain in the buttocks on hip flexion, this indicates a soft tissue lesion, such as an abscess or bursitis, under the gluteus maximus muscle.

ROM of internal and external rotation can be done with knees extended if it is not possible to have the patient perform the test in the sitting position with their knees flexed. The patella can be used as a bony landmark when examining for external and internal rotation with the patient's knees extended. Hoppenfeld[5] suggests that the therapist can examine for anteversion and retroversion of the hip with the patient lying in the supine position in which one sights down the extremity (Fig. 2-4). In the normal condition the patient's foot is

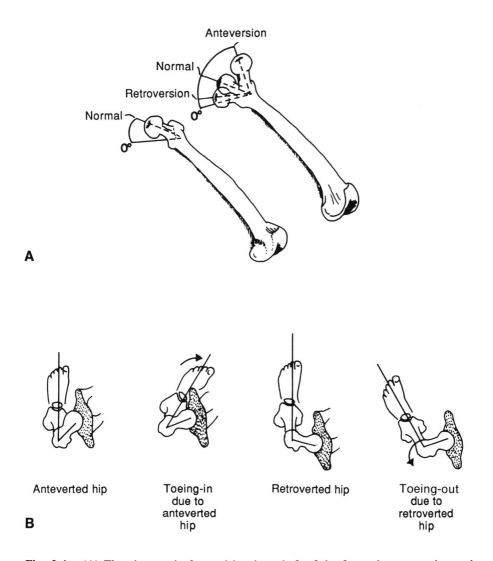

Fig. 2-4. (A) The changes in femoral head to shaft of the femur in anteversion and retroversion. (B) This same information in relation to the patella and foot position.

slightly externally rotated in relationship to the femur as one sights down across the femur and across the patella. In the anteverted hip there is a tendency for the foot to be either in the upright neutral position or inverted with the patella then being internally rotated in relationship to the greater trochanter and the head of the femur. In the retroverted hip, the opposite is true; the hip appears to be toed out and the patella would then be facing outward as well as the foot facing outward in relationship to sighting across the greater trochanter of the hip (Fig. 2-4).

In infants, with the child supine with knees extended, normal external rotation would allow you to turn the feet out and in without difficulty. Limited external rotation or excess internal rotation is typical of the anteverted hip. Again, the opposite is true with hip retroversion, in which excess external rotation and limited internal rotation is typical

Neurologic Examination

Hoppenfeld[5] uses the convention of manual muscle testing and sensation testing as being part of the neurologic examination of the musculoskeletal system. This is a very useful convention because it focuses the examiner's attention not just on manual muscle function testing, but also on the nerve root and peripheral nerve innervation of the muscles being tested.

I assume that users of this text are already well aware of the typical rating systems for manual muscle testing, so these will not be discussed. In many instances the initial manual muscle examination of the patient is a gross one to see if patients can perform the basic movements, and then if they can, whether they can take resistance to the movement. As areas of weakness are discovered, more specific manual muscle testing procedures are done.

Primary *hip flexors* are the iliopsoas muscles, innervated by the L1 and L2 nerve roots. These are usually tested in the sitting position. *Hip abductors* are tested in the side-lying position. The primary abductor is the gluteus medius muscle, innervated by the L5 and S1 nerve roots and the superior gluteal nerve. The gluteus medius muscle is assisted by the gluteus minimus muscle. Also in the sidelying position, the *adductor* muscle group is tested with the normal uninvolved leg supported by the examiner in the abducted position while the person adducts from the table towards their uninvolved leg. The primary adductor is the adductor longus, innervated by L2, L3, and L4 (obturator) nerve and assisted by the adductor brevis, adductor magnus, pectineus, and gracilis muscles.

The other major muscle group in this area to be tested contains the hip extensors. The primary extensor is the gluteus maximus, innervated by the inferior gluteal nerve (L5 + S1 nerve roots). Secondary extensors are the hamstring muscles, innervated by the sciatic nerve (L5 + S1).

In addition to the muscles around the hip joint, a complete examination should test the primary function of the hamstrings and the quadriceps muscles as well as the trunk extensor and trunk flexors. It is important for the examiner to note when the standard manual muscle test positions could not be followed and to document in what position the patient was tested so that as the patient achieves the normal testing positions in future manual muscle tests, the examiner can account for any discrepancies.

For sensation testing the physical therapist should be aware of the dermatomal nerve root as well as the peripheral nerve supplies. The hip region sensory examination includes not just the buttocks and thigh, but also the lower abdomen and trunk. The area of primary supply of the inferior femoral cutaneous, lateral femoral cutaneous, and posterior femoral cutaneous nerves should be examined. The most common examination for sensation is done by pinprick, often with a pin-wheel, which improves objectivity and is easier to manage than a pin. In addition the area can be tested for touch and for thermal modalities. Testing for thermal modalities is usually only done when the patient complains of a loss of a specific thermal modality, and in this region that seems rather unlikely. In the neurologic portion of the examination it is important to compare patients' sensory loss distributions for peripheral nerve versus dermatomes and to compare this information to the distribution of muscle weakness, if any. In addition, when the patient is describing changes in sensation the examiner should determine whether these are related to problems with the sciatic nerve, a common cause of complaints of sensory change in the posterior buttock and thigh.

Special Tests

A variety of special tests can be performed in the examination of the hip area. An important one is the Trendelenburg test for weakness of the abductors of the hip, specifically the gluteus medius muscle. The patient is asked to stand on one leg at a time; the Trendelenburg sign is positive if when standing on the involved leg the pelvis on the side opposite stays in the neutral position or drops (Fig. 2-5). Also, the Trendelenburg characteristic can be seen during walking if the patient lurches to counteract the imbalance caused by his descending hip so that the lurch is on the side of the involvement or gluteus medius weakness.

Tests for leg length discrepancy may be very important as part of the hip examination. There are two common methods for measuring leg length discrepancies. The first measurement is known as the true leg length (Fig. 2-6). With the patient lying in the supine position the examiner places the legs so that they are in approximately the same position and measures the distance from the anterior superior iliac spine to the medial malleolus of both legs. It is important for the examiner to realize that while he is measuring from one fixed point to another, he is palpating for bony landmarks through soft tissues. The examiner should therefore arrange to do the measurement so that the same hand positioning and measurement is used for both legs. One suggested technique is to palpate for the anterior superior iliac spine, slide distally from this slightly into the depression, and then measure from this point to the tip of the medial malleolus. It is

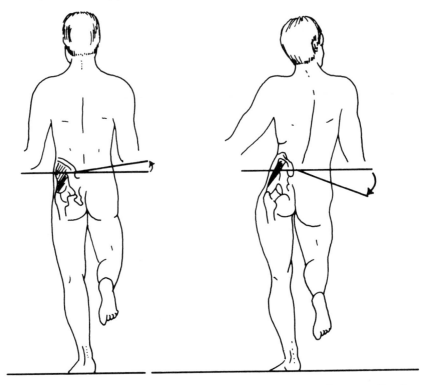

Fig. 2-5. The hip dropping on the side opposite weakness of the gluteus medius demonstrates a positive Trendelenburg sign.

important to be sure that the course of the tape follows the same route for both legs.

  The second method measures the apparent leg length discrepancy. It should be done only after the true leg length discrepancy test has been performed. The

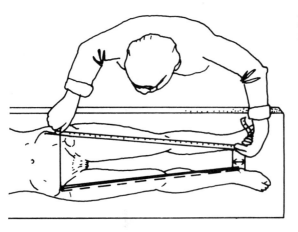

Fig. 2-6. The method for measuring "true" leg length.

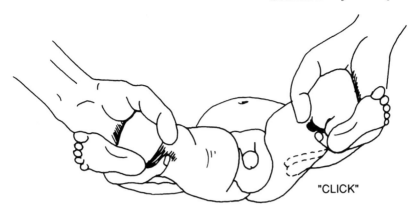

"CLICK"

Fig. 2-7. The examination method of hip flexion, abduction and external rotation of the hip joints of an infant for congenital dislocation. The test is positive if a click occurs (referred to as the Ortolani click).

patient continues to lie in a supine position and the measurement is made from the umbilicus to the tip of the medial malleolus of both legs. If these distances are not equal, this indicates an apparent leg length discrepancy, which is most likely caused by some factor resulting in pelvic obliquity, to which the examiner should then direct attention. Patients can also have tibial and femoral leg length discrepancies. These are most easily measured when the patient lies in the supine position with knees slightly flexed. For tibial shortening the examiner looks at the patient from the foot of the table to see if both knees are at the same height. For femoral length discrepancy the examiner looks at the patient from the side to see if both knees are at the same position.

Other special tests of the hip joint are related to examination of the infant. In the newborn, both hips can be equally flexed, abducted, and externally rotated without producing a click. However, when this maneuver is performed in a child with a congenital dislocation, a click is detected; this has been named the Ortolani click after the person who described this procedure (Fig. 2-7). In addition to this test for congenital dislocation there is also the "telescoping" test in which the examiner grasps the infant by the tibia with the knee slightly flexed and gently distracts and compresses the hip, looking for easy movement of the entire femur while at the same time palpating over the area of the greater trochanter (Fig. 2-8). The Barlow test may also be used. In this test the thumb of the examiner is placed on the inner aspect of the thigh. The hip is abducted and downward pressure exerted, pushing the thigh toward the examining table.

Another important test to be carried out in the hip region is the Fabre test in which the patient is placed in flexion, abduction, and external rotation and pressure is applied downward over the knee, stressing the hip joint. In patients with hip problems, pain will usually be produced in the area of the inguinal region or lateral aspect of the hip. If the patient notes discomfort over the sacroiliac joint, the examiner should conduct further tests of sacroiliac joint dysfunction.

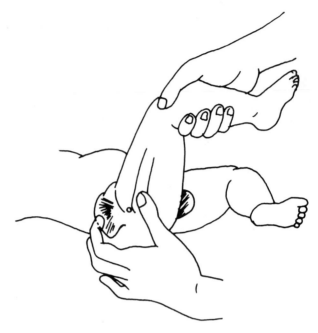

Fig. 2-8. Procedure for performing the "telescoping" examination of the hip of an infant.

Examination of Related Areas

Since there is an intimate relationship between the lumbosacral region and the buttocks, particularly in regard to dermatomal and nerve root problems, any examination of the hip joint should include a brief examination of the lumbar spine. The details of the examination of the lumbar spine are beyond the scope of this particular book and chapter, but there are several sources of information regarding this examination, and certainly a simple examination of ROM of the lumbar spine, straight leg raising tests, and a search for evidence of nerve root problems in the lower extremity by sensory and reflex testing would be the minimum that would be required.

Other Information of Importance

It is difficult when looking at the hip region not to look at the entire lower extremity, particularly in relation to its vascular status: the arterial system (by checking pulses in the extremity) and the veins (by searching for varicosities or other vascular problems).

It is important for the physical therapist to look at available x-rays of the area since the hip joint is deep and not amenable to direct examination. The physical therapist should also look at observational gait characteristics, which may be one of the first things done in examining the hip (see Ch. 9). Keep in mind that many of the observational gait characteristics represent specific weaknesses of muscle groups around the hip. The example used in this chapter was the Trendelenburg sign and the Trendelenburg gait characteristic. Also, it is important to remember that the hip is a major weightbearing joint and as such affects the attitude and posture of several other areas of the body (see Ch. 9). Obviously, changes at the hip joint affect posture at both the knee and the ankle as well as posture of the segments above the hip.

Since many of the patients who have hip joint dysfunctions are among the elderly patient group, it is important for the physical therapist to have some understanding of the special problems and characteristics of dealing with this patient population. It is important to examine unexplained weakness around the hip joint in whatever way leads to the most important information. Femoral nerve compressions can and do occur, and therefore nerve conduction velocity testing and electromyographic (EMG) testing can lead to important information. Nerve root compression also can cause problems relating to weakness around the hip joint; testing for this can provide important information in selected patients. Finally, one should always relate the material gathered during the examination to the final use of this material in decision making about the patient. One of the more important characteristics of the base line information derived from the first examination of the patient is how this can help us to reevaluate the patient, particularly in regard to successive treatment planning.

When the examination is finished, the therapist should be able to hypothesize the cause of the patient's difficulties. A responsibility of the physical therapist in a direct access scheme is to either solve the patient's problems or to refer the patient to someone who can.[3,4] Please see Appendix 2-2 for a hip algorithm that may help with this area; if using the HOAC system as part of this strategy, it will be clear when referral or consultation is needed for both treatment planning and for assessing failure when patients do not progress satisfactorily. One of the most challenging aspects of examining a patient is the use made of the information derived from the examination in treatment planning and future decision making about the patient.

REFERENCES

1. Delitto A: Subjective measures and clinical decision making. Phys Ther 69:585, 1989
2. Jette AN: Measuring subjective clinical outcomes. Phys Ther 69:580, 1989
3. Rothstein JM: On defining subjective and objective measurements. Phys Ther 69:577, 1989
4. Echternach JL, Rothstein JM: Hypothesis oriented algorithms. Phys Ther 69: 559, 1989
5. Hoppenfeld S: Physical examination of the hip and pelvis. pp. 143. In Physical Examination of the Spine and Extremities. Appleton-Century-Crofts, East Norwalk, CT, 1976

6. Saudek CE: The Hip. p. 365. In Gould JA, Davies JG (Eds.): Orthopedic and Sports Physical Therapy. CV Mosby, St. Louis, 1985

7. Adams CJ: The Hip Region. pp. 311. In Outline of Orthopaedics. 9th Ed. Churchill Livingstone, New York, 1981

8. Maitland GF: Lower limb. p. 203. In Peripheral Manipulation, 2 Ed. Butterworths, London, 1980

9. Woerman AL: Evaluation and treatment of dysfunction in the lumbar pelvic hip complex. p. 403. In Donatelli R, Wooden MJ (Eds.): Orthopaedic Physical Therapy. Churchill Livingstone, New York, 1989

10. Cyriax J: The buttock and hip. p. 595–621. In Textbook on Orthopedic Medicine, Vol. 1: Diagnosis of Soft Tissue Lesions. 7th Ed. Baillier, Tindall, London, 1978

Standard Hip Region Evaluation as Performed at Old Dominion University Program in Physical Therapy

I. **Objective**
    A. To state in writing the components of an acceptable hip region evaluation
    B. To assist in developing proficiency in performing an evaluation of hip region problems

II. **Conducting the Evaluation**
    A. Subjective
        1. *History:* Obtain from chart and patient. Include date of onset, circumstances of present complaint, prior history, previous treatment including surgical, use of appliances, gait aides
        2. Subjective information from patient
            a. General: Chief complaint, pain—type and location. Is problem getting worse or better?
            b. Specific to hip: Rest pain/weightbearing and activity pain
    B. Objective
        1. *Observation:* Is pelvis level? Inspect buttock and thigh region for atrophy, asymmetry, swelling, obvious leg length discrepancy. Foot position standing—rotated?
        2. *Palpation:* Tenderness, nodules, etc. in inguinal region, femoral triangle, greater trochanter, ischial tuberosity, SI joint,

pubis–spasm of large muscle; masses of gluteals, adductors, iliopsoas area, deeper muscles, e.g., piriformis region

3. *Evaluate ROM*
   a. Hip flexion, abduction, adduction, internal and external rotation. Where does pain occur? During what part of range—active vs. passive ROM? Clicks, crepitus noted?
   b. Special tests: straight leg raising, hip flexor tightness (Thomas position), iliotibial band tightness (Ober position), Fabere
4. *Gait:* Observe for Trendelenburg, antalgic gait, uneven steps, other gait deviations—toe in, toe out
5. *Manual muscle testing:* Hip motions, positioning important for extensor, abduction, rotation
6. *Measure leg lengths:* ASIS to medial malleolus, umbilicus to medial malleolus; observe tibial lengths with knees bent. Confirm leg length with standing test of pelvic tilt and amount needed to level the pelvis
7. *Neurologic evaluation*
   a. Radiating pain—sciatic nerve and nerve root compressions vs. other causes
   b. Dysthesias and paresthesias
   c. Sensory loss—peripheral nerve vs. dermatome
   d. Distribution of muscle weakness
8. *Miscellaneous*
   Further evaluation done as need arises. Consider requests for additional information.
   a. X-rays: hip joint, anteroposterior and rotated views, pelvis if related to pubic area, ischium, sacroiliac joints
   b. Check femoral pulse bilaterally
   c. Look at varicosities, other vascular signs
   d. electromyography nerve conduction velocity if femoral nerve, vs. nerve root problems
   e. Patient's mental status—cooperative vs. emotionally upset, traumatic incident, or secondary gain factors

APPENDIX 2-2
Hip Pain Algorithm

Hip Examination & Initial Evaluation

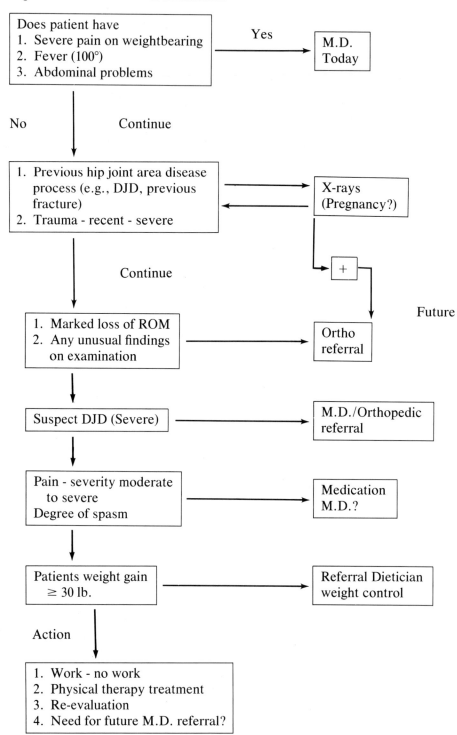

3 | Biomechanics of the Hip

Carol A. Oatis

The hip joint is a ball-and-socket joint with a twofold function: to position the lower extremity in space and to bear weight. Its structure allows mobility without sacrificing stability. This chapter presents the specializations of the hip joint affecting its mobility and weightbearing capacity.

ALIGNMENT

Alignment of the hip joint affects its weightbearing capabilities as well as the motion available at the joint. Consideration must be given to the individual positions of the acetabulum and femoral head and then to their relative positions. The effects of malalignment must also be considered.

The acetabulum is positioned on the lateral aspect of the pelvis facing laterally, anteriorly, and inferiorly. The femoral head faces medially, anteriorly, and superiorly.[1] Thus, in the anatomic position the fovea, or pit, of the head of the femur is directed slightly toward the anterior and superior aspect of the acetabulum. The acetabulum then forms a roof and posterior wall for the femoral head (Fig. 3-1).

The orientation of the femoral head and acetabulum has two effects, the first on the static forces applied to the hip joint, and the second on the motions of the hip. The femoral head and acetabulum orientation causes the contact force between the femur and acetabulum to be high in the anterosuperior region of the joint.[2] Pauwels[3] and Maquet[4] reported that during quiet standing, the joint reaction force is oriented in a more vertical direction than the femoral head, which tends to produce a bending moment through the femoral neck. The bending moment produces compressive forces on the inferior surface of the femoral neck and tensile forces on the superior surface (Fig. 3-2).

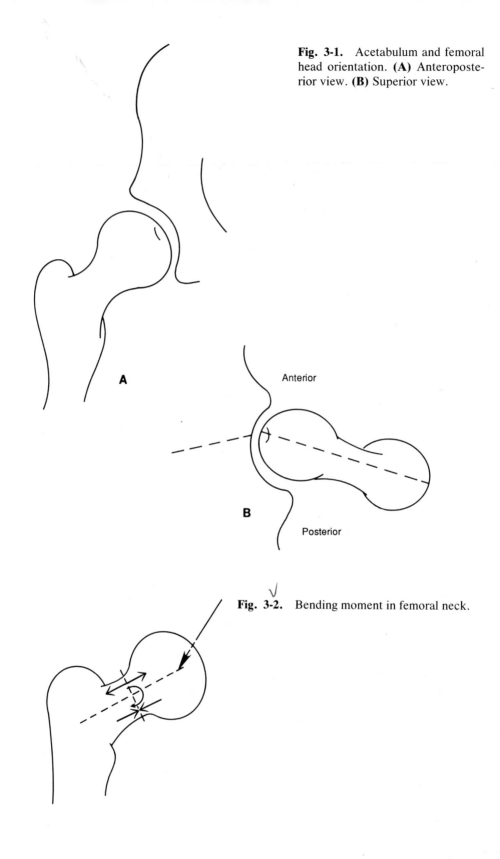

Fig. 3-1. Acetabulum and femoral head orientation. **(A)** Anteroposterior view. **(B)** Superior view.

A

Anterior

B

Posterior

Fig. 3-2. Bending moment in femoral neck.

Several investigators have reported that the trabecular bone of the femoral neck is arranged in arrays that reinforce the femoral neck to sustain the joint reaction force. A medial bundle of cancellous bone originates from the medial cortex of the femoral shaft and extends upward onto the weightbearing surface of the femoral head. This column of cancellous bone is parallel to the joint reaction force and appears to sustain the neck against the joint reaction force. A lateral array of cancellous bone runs from the base of the greater trochanter and lateral cortex of the neck, intersects the medial array within the femoral head, and continues into the inferior aspect of the head. Maquet[4] noted that this bundle is parallel to the tensile stresses in the femoral neck, while Frankel and Pugh[5] stated that it protects the neck against the compressive forces generated by the hip abductor muscles. Further stress analysis appears necessary to identify definitively the role of the lateral bundle of trabecular bone. However, it seems that its highly organized arrangement reflects its task of reinforcing the femoral neck against the unique loads applied to it.

The second effect of femoral head-acetabular orientation affects the motion of the hip joint. Because the anterior aspect of the femoral head is somewhat exposed in the anatomic position, the joint has much more flexibility in flexion than in extension. Specific ranges of motion are considered in more detail later in this chapter.

To achieve the relative orientation of the acetabulum and femur described above, the femur must develop a specific shape with characteristic orientations in the frontal and transverse planes. The frontal plane shape is described as coxa vara or valga, and the transverse plane shape as anteversion or retroversion. Each is addressed separately in the following section.

In the frontal plane, the angle of inclination of the femoral neck on the shaft is generally accepted to be approximately 125°.[1,6] However, Yoshioka et al.[7] found a mean angle of 131° from 32 cadaveric specimens. An increase in the angle between the shaft and head is known as coxa valga. In this alignment, the femoral head is directed more superiorly in the acetabulum. Maquet[4] reported many biomechanical effects of this alignment based on earlier studies by Pauwels. First, photoelastic studies revealed that in coxa valga, the joint reaction force at the hip is almost parallel to the femoral shaft. The cancellous bone appears to develop in straight columns also parallel to the femoral neck. These phenomena suggest that the femoral neck sustains mostly compressive forces in the presence of coxa valga (Fig. 3-3). In addition, Maquet[4] noted that a coxa valga deformity shortens the moment arm of the abductor muscles, which would decrease their mechanical advantage (Fig. 3-4). Consequently, the abductors would have to contract more vigorously to stabilize the pelvis, causing an increase in the joint reaction force. Finally, Maquet[4] also stated that coxa valga results in a lateral displacement of the joint reaction force and reduces the weightbearing surface. The increased joint reaction force with a concomitant decrease in weightbearing area will increase the stress (force per unit area) on the particular surfaces. In addition, the displacement of the joint reaction force may result in forces applied across joint surfaces not specialized to sustain such loads. In other words, a coxa valga deformity causes several deleterious altera-

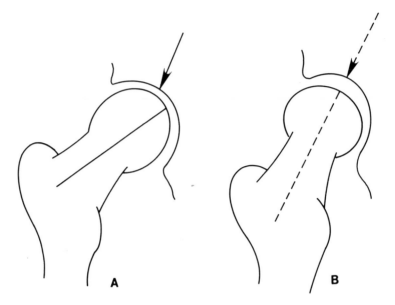

Fig. 3-3. Effects of coxa valga. **(A)** Normal frontal plane alignment. **(B)** Coxa valga with joint reaction force parallel to femoral neck.

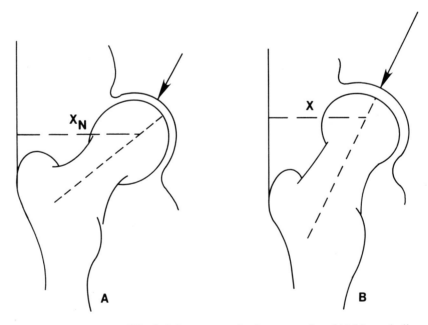

Fig. 3-4. Moment arm (X) of abductor muscles in coxa valga. **(A)** Normal alignment (X_N). **(B)** Coxa valga ($X < X_N$).

tions in joint mechanics that may result in degenerative changes in the articular surfaces.

Coxa vara is the deformity of the femoral head-shaft orientation in which the angle is less than normal. Some of its mechanical effects are opposite those of coxa valga. A coxa vara deformity moves the trochanter laterally, away from the pelvis, effectively lengthening the moment arm of the abductor muscles (Fig. 3-5).[4] In contrast to coxa valga, this position improves the mechanical advantage of the abductors so that they can contract *less vigorously* to produce adequate force to stabilize the pelvis, thus reducing the joint reaction force. This positive effect of coxa vara has been applied in the utilization of various osteotomies of the femur for the treatment of osteoarthrosis of the hip joint[8] or aseptic necrosis of the femoral head.[9] It has also been reported that the joint reaction force is displaced medially in coxa vara, creating increased compressive forces medially and increased tensile forces laterally.[4] These changes are reportedly reflected in increased arching of the arrays of trabecular bone in the femoral neck. However, coxa vara effectively widens the pelvis, so in order to keep the knees and feet together as in normal posture, the angle of the femur, and hence the angle of the knee, in the frontal plane will increase. These changes could again present potential problems for the rest of the lower extremity. While the effects of coxa vara appear to be less deleterious than those of coxa valga, they do emphasize the dependence of the hip joint mechanics on femoral alignment.

The effects of coxa vara and valga demonstrate the principles underlying the mechanism of slipped capital femoral epiphysis. While the adult femur has a neck-shaft angle of approximately 125°, the developing femur demonstrates

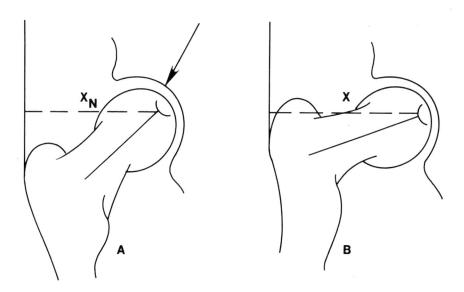

Fig. 3-5. Moment arm (X) of abductor muscles in coxa vara. **(A)** Normal alignment (X_N). **(B)** Coxa vara ($X > X_N$).

considerably more coxa valga, which gradually decreases to normal throughout growth.[10] Failure of the epiphyseal plate occurs as a result of shear forces, which are forces applied parallel to the surface of the growth plate.[11] Maquet[4] reported that the joint reaction force should be perpendicular to the growth plate, which would result in no shear component. However, Pauwels[3] suggested that as the coxa valga of the growing femur decreases, the capital epiphysis may no longer be perpendicular to the joint reaction force. The reaction force can then be broken into two components, one that is perpendicular to the plate and is compressive, and one that is parallel to the plate and is shearing (Fig. 3-6). If the joint reaction force is excessive, which occurs in obesity, or if it is aligned so that the shear component is too great, the shearing force will exceed the strength of the epiphysis in shear and the plate will fail, or slip.[11] Again, understanding the mechanics of the normal joint provides a basis for understanding pathology within the hip joint.

Femoral alignment in the transverse plane also influences the mechanics of the hip joint. In normal development, the proximal femur undergoes a twisting or torsion on the distal femur. Anteversion is defined as the anterior position of the axis through the femoral condyles.[12,13] Normal femoral anteversion in the adult is approximately 12° to 15°. Retroversion indicates a femoral neck axis that is parallel or posterior to the condylar axis (Fig. 3-7). Yoshioka et al.[7] reported wide variability in femoral anteversion in 32 embalmed femoral specimens. Pizzutillo et al.[12] reported a means of 32° of anteversion at birth that decreased to 15° by 16 years of age based on 1,190 clinical examinations.

Excessive anteversion directs the femoral head toward the anterior aspect of the acetabulum when the femoral condyles are aligned in their normal orienta-

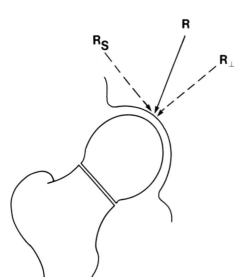

Fig. 3-6. Shear (R_s) and compression ($R_\perp$) components of joint reaction force (R) with epiphyseal plate.

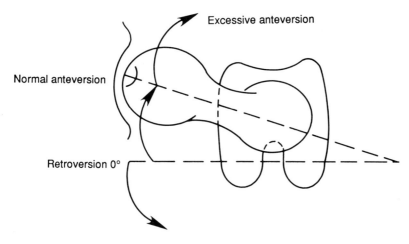

Fig. 3-7. Transverse plane alignment of the hip joint.

tion in the frontal plane. Consequently, internal rotation of the femur is required to seat the femoral head normally in the acetabulum. Subjects with excessive anteversion usually have much more hip internal rotation range of motion than external rotation and gravitate to the typical "frog-sitting" posture as a position of comfort. Because the femoral head can assume an optimal position in the acetabulum only with internal rotation of the femur, the common clinical manifestation of excessive anteversion is excessive in-toeing. However, compensatory external tibial torsion that usually occurs in the first 5 to 7 years of life often eliminates the in-toeing, thus eliminating the clinical expression of the excessive anteversion.[12] However, it should not be assumed that the elimination of the clinical expression of the deformity implies an elimination of the hip deformity. Pizzutillo et al.[12] reported no change in the angle of anteversion with standard treatment such as shoe wedges, twister cables, or Denis Browne splints or with no treatment at all, although many subjects had indeed lost the in-toeing gait. These researchers advocated no intervention unless functional problems develop. They characterized the subjects who require surgical intervention as those who demonstrate little compensatory tibial torsion and have limited hip external rotation range of motion. The effects of the compensatory tibial torsion of the knee joint or on the mechanics of the foot and ankle cannot be covered in this chapter. Suffice it to say that femoral alignment in the transverse plane, like the alignment in the frontal plane, can have profound effects on the mechanics of not only the hip joint but also the entire lower extremity.

HIP JOINT RANGE OF MOTION

Normal hip joint range of motion has been reported frequently. Miller[14] has discussed the limitations of the standards of normal range of motion. He reported wide variability in the normal ranges reported by many investigators.

Table 3-1. Values of Normal Ranges of Motion of the Hip Reported in the Literature

Motion	Miller[a]	Frankel & Pugh[b]
Flexion	100–130°	140°
Extension	10–50°	15°
Abduction	40–55°	30°
Adduction	0–45°	<25°
External rotation	36–50°	90°
Internal rotation	30–47°	70°

[a] Range of normal values of range of motion as presented by Miller.[14]
[b] Values of normal ranges reported by Frankel and Pugh.[5]

The range of these normal joint excursions for the hip joint as reported by Miller is presented in Table 3-1. Also included in this table are values reported by Frankel and Pugh.[5] The wide disagreement among researchers is difficult to explain because, as Miller[14] points out so clearly, few include with their norms data on the population from which the numbers were derived or on the methodology used to acquire the results. Thus, the clinician must be cautioned to use standard values of normalcy with reserve; that is, these values provide some perspective, but no single value appears to have risen as the "gold standard" of normal.

The relative position of the pelvis and the femur determine hip joint position. Because the lower extremity often functions as a closed kinetic chain in which the proximal segment moves on a fixed distal segment, the clinician must be able to identify hip positions when the pelvis moves rather than when the femur does. For example, with the femur fixed, an anterior pelvic tilt puts the hip in relative flexion. In single limb support with the stance limb fixed, the pelvis drops on the unsupported side and causes relative adduction of the stance hip. Finally, in the transverse plane, during single-limb stance on the right, the pelvis rotates forward on the contralateral, or left, side, putting the stance hip in relative internal rotation (Fig. 3-8).

HIP JOINT MECHANICS

No chapter on the biomechanics of the hip is complete without a discussion of the mechanics of single-limb stance. This particular event has generated much interest for two reasons. First, single-limb support occurs twice with every stride and therefore happens thousands of times a day for the normal individual. Second, analysis of the forces sustained by a subject in a single-limb stance allows the reader to appreciate the significant loads that the hip endures during a relatively sedate activity. Further analysis or mental interpolation can provide a perspective that reveals the enormous loads that the hip must sustain in such vigorous activities as running or jumping.

The basic task in single-limb stance is to balance the weight of the head,

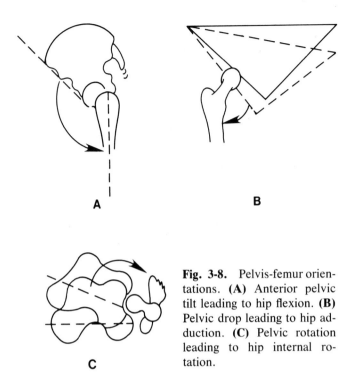

A   **B**

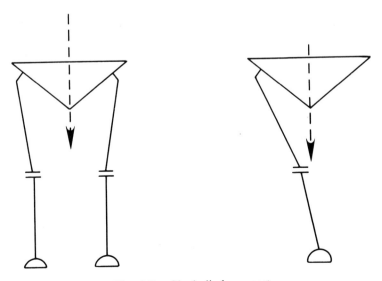

Fig. 3-8. Pelvis-femur orientations. **(A)** Anterior pelvic tilt leading to hip flexion. **(B)** Pelvic drop leading to hip adduction. **(C)** Pelvic rotation leading to hip internal rotation.

C

arms, trunk, and opposite leg (HATL) on the stance limb. To maintain an upright position, a line through the center of mass of the HATL weight must fall through the base of support, which is the stance foot. To achieve this position, the subject must shift laterally so that the stance hip is adducted (Fig. 3-9). The

Fig. 3-9.   Single-limb support.

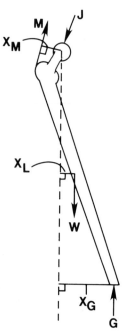

Fig. 3-10. Free-body diagram of the stance limb.

weight of the HATL tends to fall to the unsupported side, and the abductor muscles on the stance side must pull the weight back toward the stance limb so that the HATL weight is balanced on top of the stance limb.

To analyze the single-limb stance, two basic questions must be answered: What is the force required of the abductor muscles to balance the load of the HATL? What is the load exerted on the femoral head during single-limb support? A free-body diagram of the stance limb allows visualization of all the forces on the stance limb (Fig. 3-10). The HATL weight is not included independently on the femoral head, but is represented in some unknown proportion in the joint reaction force, J. The ground reaction force, G, on the other hand, directly reflects the effect of body weight on the stance limb.

Application of the conditions of static equilibrium allows calculation of the muscle and joint reaction forces:

$$\Sigma Fx = 0$$
$$\Sigma Fy = 0 \qquad (1)$$
$$\Sigma FM = 0$$

$$J = J_x{}^2 + J_y{}^2 \qquad (5)$$

Moment equilibrium yields the following:

$$\Sigma M: M_G - M_L - M_M = 0 \qquad (2)$$

where M_g, M_L, and M_M are the moments due to the ground reaction force, weight of the stance limb, and force of the abductor muscles, respectively. Moments are force times the perpendicular distance from the force to the point of rotation, that is, force times its moment arm. Note that the joint reaction force causes no moment because it is applied at the point of rotation and therefore has a zero moment arm. Inclusion of the moment arms yields:

$$\Sigma M: (G \times X_G) - (W \times X_L) - (M \times X_M) = 0 \qquad (3)$$

Since all but M, the force of the abductors, can be measured or estimated, the equation can be solved for the force of the abductors. The solution reveals that the force of the abductors required to maintain upright posture is approximately two times body weight. Application of the criteria of force equilibrium allows solution of the joint reaction force:

$$\Sigma F_x: M_x + J_x = 0 \text{ and} \qquad (4)$$
$$\Sigma F_y: M_y + J_y - L - G = 0$$

Note that because L and G are weights, they always are vertical and directed downward and therefore are negative and have no x component. The x and y components of the known forces are determined by simple trigonometric calculations. The total joint reaction force is calculated by using the Pythagorean theorem:

$$J = J_x^2 + J_y^2 \qquad (5)$$

Solving these equations will reveal that the joint reaction force is approximately 2.5 to 2.75 times body weight.

Why are such large forces generated by the abductor muscles and why does the femoral head sustain such loads? The answers lie in a comparison of the moment arm of the abductor muscles with the moment arm of the ground reaction force. Because the subject must keep the center of gravity over the stance foot, the subject must shift the pelvis laterally, moving the point of rotation (the hip joint) laterally away from the stance foot, thus lengthening the moment arm of the ground reaction force (Fig. 3-11). Consequently, the moment arm of the ground reaction force is much longer than that of the abductor muscles, and the muscles must exert a very large force to counteract this difference.

It is this difference in moment arms that explains the usefulness of a cane when used in the contralateral hand. One of the roles of a cane is to lower the load on the stance limb. To lower the hip joint reaction force, the force of the abductors must be reduced. Patients with weakness of the abductor muscles accomplish this by shifting their body weight laterally toward the stance limb during stance on the weak side, thus moving the center of mass closer to the point of rotation and decreasing or even eliminating the moment arm of the ground reaction force (Fig. 3-12). However, when a subject uses a cane,

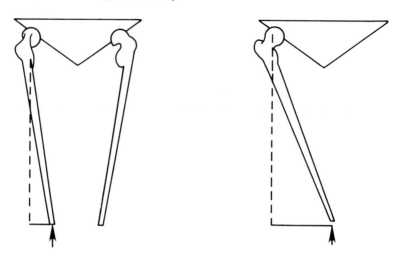

Fig. 3-11.   Lateral shift of pelvis in single-limb support.

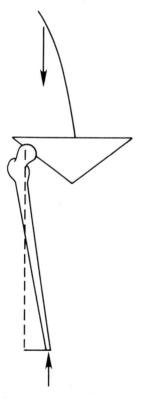

Fig. 3-12.   Gluteus medius limp.

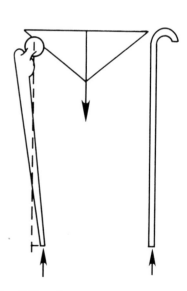

Fig. 3-13.   Stance during single-limb support with the use of a cane.

the need for the shift is eliminated. The cane widens the base of support and allows the subject to stand erect with the center of mass falling between the stance foot and the cane. This allows the subject to stand with the stance foot almost directly under the hip joint, decreasing the moment arm of the ground reaction force substantially and consequently decreasing the force exerted by the hip abductors (Fig. 3-13). The cane is not so important as a load-bearing device but rather as a device that allows erect posture. Some estimates suggest that a subject who applies only one-sixth body weight can reduce the joint reaction force by almost 50 percent.[15] Thus, the reader would be well-advised to consider the advice proffered by William Blount in 1956: "Don't throw away the cane."[16]

SUMMARY

The hip joint is designed to provide both mobility and stability. Both roles are influenced by the relative alignment of the pelvis and femur and particularly the internal alignment of the femur. In addition, the forces sustained by the hip joint are a function of the subject's standing posture. These forces are substantial even under static conditions, approximately more than twice body weight.

REFERENCES

1. Nordin N, Frankel VH: Biomechanics of the hip. p. 149. In Frankel VH, Nordin N (eds): Basic Biomechanics of the Skeletal System. Lea & Febiger, Philadelphia, 1980
2. Afoke NYP, Byers PD, Hutton WC: Contact pressures in the human hip joint. J Bone Joint Surg 69B:536, 1987
3. Pauwels F: Biomechanics of the Normal and Diseased Hip. Springer-Verlag, Berlin, 1976
4. Maquet PGJ: Biomechanics of the Hip as Applied to Osteoarthritis and Related Conditions. Springer-Verlag, Berlin, 1985
5. Frankel VH, Pugh JW: Biomechanics of the hip. p. 115. In Tronzo RG (ed): Surgery of the Hip Joint. Vol. 1. Springer-Verlag, Berlin, 1984
6. Kapandji IA: The Physiology of the Joints. Vol. 2. Lower Limb. Churchill Livingstone, Edinburgh, 1970
7. Yoshioka Y, Siu D, Cooke TDV: Anatomy and Functional Axes of the Femur. J Bone Joint Surg 69A:873, 1987
8. Goldie IF, Dumbleton JH: Intertrochanteric osteotomy of the femur. p. 72. In Black J, Dumbleton JH (eds): Clinical Biomechanics. A Case History Approach. Churchill Livingstone, New York, 1981
9. Lunceford EM, Weinstein AM, Koeneman JB: Femoral head arthroplasty for aseptic necrosis. p. 140. In Black J, Dumbleton JH (eds): Clinical Biomechanics. A Case History Approach. Churchill Livingstone, New York, 1981
10. Goss CM (ed): Anatomy of the Human Body by Henry Gray, FRS. Lea & Febiger, Philadelphia, 1973
11. Chung SMK, Hirata TT: Multiple pin repair of the slipped capital femoral epiphysis. p. 94. In Black J, Dumbleton JH (eds): Clinical Biomechanics. A Case History Approach. Churchill Livingstone, New York, 1981

12. Pizzutillo PT, MacEwen GD, Shands AR: Anteversion of the femur. In Tonzo RG (ed): Surgery of the Hip Joint. Vol. 1. Springer-Verlag, New York, 1984
13. Lausten GS, Jorgensen F, Boesen J: Measurement of anteversion of the femoral neck, ultrasound and CT compared. J Bone Joint Surg 71B:237, 1989
14. Miller PJ: Assessment of joint motion. p. 103. In Rothstein JM (ed): Measurement in Physical Therapy. Churchill Livingstone, New York, 1985
15. Benedek GB, Villars FMH: Physics with Illustrative Examples from Medicine and Biology. Vol. 1. Mechanics. Addison-Wesley, Reading, PA, 1973
16. Blount W: Don't throw away the cane. J Bone Joint Surg 38A:695, 1956

4 | Common Pathologic Problems of the Hip

Curtis V. Spear, Jr.

The hip joint is an enarthrodial or ball-and-socket joint formed by the head or proximal portion of the femur and the cup-shaped cavity of the acetabulum of the pelvis. This joint is prevented from dislocating by several very strong ligaments, the strongest of which is the iliofemoral ligament. The iliofemoral ligament, the strongest ligament in the body, is placed on stretch by any attempt to extend the femur beyond a straight line with the trunk. This ligament is the chief agent in maintaining the erect position without muscular fatigue. Hyperextension of the hip joint causes the center of gravity of the trunk to come behind the center of rotation of the hip joint and, therefore, is prevented by tension in the iliofemoral ligament.

ARTHRITIS

The national health interview survey has shown that each year approximately 10 percent of the population or 23 million Americans have arthritic symptoms severe enough to require medical attention or restrict their activity.

Osteoarthritis

Osteoarthritis is the term used by most clinicians in the United States. Osteoarthrosis, degenerative joint disease, degenerative arthritis, hypertrophic arthritis, or wear-and-tear arthritis is the most common form of arthritis. This form of arthritis is caused by wear and destruction of the hyaline cartilage,

51

which is the type that covers the ends of the bones where joints are formed. The incidence of this type of arthritis increases with age and is seen in 80 percent of men and 89 percent of women after the age of 75. It is interesting that before the age of 45, men are more commonly affected than women. After the age of 45, women are more commonly affected.[1] Many patients with early osteoarthritis have no associated symptoms or disability. Information from Haynes One (Health and Nutritional Examinations, Survey One) reveals that only 50 percent of patients with radiographic evidence of severe arthritis of the hip reported pain in that area on most days during one month.[2]

Osteoarthritis of the hip occurs more commonly late in life and has an unknown cause. Osteoarthritis is usually slowly progressive, most frequently affecting the hands and the large weightbearing joints. It is characterized clinically by pain, limitation of motion, and deformity. Pathologically, one sees fibrillation of the hyaline cartilage, thinning of the cartilage, local areas of erosion with cartilage destruction, and subchondral bony sclerosis. Later, cysts develop under the adjacent surfaces of the joint with large outgrowths of bone, or osteophytes, along the joint margin. Intermittently, one sees inflammation of the synovium, or tissue covering, of the joint, which is usually secondary to the bony lesions. Systemic abnormalities are not seen with osteoarthritis.

There is no genetic transmission of this disease, although some believe that the type of osteoarthritis seen in the first metatarsophalangeal joints of the feet and the hand, which occurs more often in women, may be transmitted genetically, with incomplete penetrance in men.[3] Osteoarthritis can occur with certain genetic chemical abnormalities, such as alkaptonuria, ochronosis, and hemochromatosis, as well as in childhood abnormalities, such as slipped femoral capital epiphyses, Legg-Calvé-Perthes disease, and congenital dysplasia of the hip.

Osteoarthritis can also occur in patients who have had trauma to joints with a resulting irregular surface of the joint. It is thought to be more common in individuals in certain occupations, such as farmers and athletes, although this is not uniformly held to be true.[3] Osteoarthritis has been classified as both a primary and secondary condition. In primary arthritis there is no obvious etiology. In secondary arthritis a pre-existing condition causes an irregularity of the joint and, therefore, premature accelerated wear. The symptoms are the same in both cases. One type of primary arthritis usually involves several joints, commonly does not occur before the age of 35, and is of unknown etiology. Monoarticular arthritis, involving only one joint, is associated with an incongruity of the surfaces of the joint. It is secondary to mechanical derangements and can follow congenital abnormalities, infections, Legg-Calvé-Perthes disease, and fractures involving the joint.

Osteoarthritis of the hip usually occurs in older patients and is usually progressive, leading to complete destruction of the joint and requiring surgery. The point at which degenerative arthritis of the hip becomes symptomatic varies considerably from individual to individual. In the earlier stages of arthritis of the hip, the patient is aware of the joint being uncomfortable and usually notes a relationship to activity. With the passage of time, the patient may notice being unable to walk up steps or unable to step up with the involved leg. The patient may note increasing difficulty in putting on socks or stockings because of progressive stiffness of the hip. The patient may notice the presence of pain at night when moving or changing positions during sleep, as well as progressive limitation in the distance that he or she can walk and remain comfortable. During this stage, one usually notices more difficulty in carrying out routine activities associated with work and a progressive limitation in being able to participate in recreational activities. During the earlier stages, rest, heat, and oral anti-inflammatory medication is usually the only treatment necessary. Active and mild passive exercises are helpful in maintaining mobility in the joint and good muscle tone. A cane or crutches may be utilized during more painful periods. Surgical treatment is usually necessary when patients are no longer able to carry out their activities of daily living or employment.

Rheumatoid Arthritis

Rheumatoid arthritis is a systemic, inflammatory, and chronic disorder of unknown etiology. The condition is characterized by exacerbations and remissions and, ultimately, destruction of the joint surfaces and progressive disability. Women are affected two to three times more often than men. The occurrence increases with age. In women, the peak incidence is usually between the fourth and sixth decades. Recent findings suggest that genetic factors can influence the expression of the disease, possibly by their effects on the immunologic phenomenon that plays a role in its pathogenesis.[4]

The features of rheumatoid arthritis along with its typical lesions suggest an exaggeration of normal immune mechanism or hypersensitivity. In approximately 70 percent of patients, an abnormal macroglobulin or rheumatoid factor is present. This can be demonstrated by serologic tests, such as the latex and sheep cell agglutinin tests. These tests usually become positive as the disease progresses. The rheumatoid factor is not pathognomonic for the disease in that it does occur in other unrelated connective tissue diseases. The latex test, used for diagnosis of rheumatoid arthritis, detects primarily the positive rheumatoid factor, which occurs in approximately 70 percent of adult patients with rheumatoid arthritis. It is not always diagnostic of this disorder in that 5 percent of normal individuals have a positive latex test. High levels of rheumatoid factor are generally associated with more severe and active joint disease and the presence of subcutaneous rheumatoid nodules. The systemic complications of rheumatoid arthritis usually suggest a poor outcome.

The earliest findings in rheumatoid arthritis occur in synovial tissue and consist of edema, mild synovial cell proliferation, and obliteration of small blood vessels by inflammatory cells in organized thrombi. As arthritic changes progress, the synovium appears more edematous and extends into the joint cavity with slender villus projections. As inflammation progresses, destruction of the articular cartilage, ligaments, tendons, and bone is seen.

Damage from the digestants in the synovial fluid as well as the growth of granulation tissue play parts in the destruction of the joint cartilage. The most destructive element in rheumatoid arthritis is the pannus or vascular granulation-type tissue that progressively grows over the hyaline cartilage, destroying it. The pannus erodes subchondral bone at the margins of the joint and burrows beneath the cartilage to produce local areas of osteolysis, or cysts, in bone. The remaining bone in the area of the joint usually shows regional osteoporosis or thinning. With time, fibrous adhesions develop between the opposing joint surfaces with a resultant fibrous ankylosis. The fibrous ankylosis may eventually turn into bone, causing a bony ankylosing or fusion of the joint.

Even the connective tissue elements of muscles controlling the joint show involvement by the inflammatory process. The result is a disuse atrophy, fibrosis, and shortening of these muscles, leading to increased stress on the adjacent joint and at times subluxation or dislocation of the joint.

In the early phases of the disease, systemic manifestations such as malaise, weight loss, and ability fatigue are seen. The original symptoms in the hip joint are vague pain and stiffness, more commonly noted when the patient first gets up in the morning and moves inflamed joints that have tended to stiffen up during sleep. After the patient has been up and about and has limbered up, the symptoms are less noticeable. With time, the stiffness and pain become more severe and more persistent.

The usual symptoms of rheumatoid arthritis—redness, swelling, increased heat, tenderness to palpation, and atrophy of adjacent muscles—seen in the smaller joints are not seen in the hip region because of the distance from the hip joint to the skin. Protective muscle spasm may be present because of pain and inflammation in the joint. Stiffness develops fairly rapidly as the joint surface is destroyed. It is characterized by the development of a hip flexion contracture. The patient holds the hip in a flexed position and notices more difficulty in putting on shoes and socks and carrying out foot care. Although medical treatment helps to suppress the associated synovitis, motion once lost from joint destruction is generally not regained. Approximately 30 percent of patients with rheumatoid arthritis have minimal symptoms and do not consult a physician for treatment.

Active exercise of the hip joint within the limits of pain is important in preserving joint motion and maintaining good muscle tone. Physical therapy, often initiated in a hospital setting, should be done at regular intervals on an outpatient basis to minimize muscle atrophy and contractures. Patient motivation is an important factor with any exercise program. If the patient reaches a point where pain is significantly interfering with the activities of daily living and occupational requirements, surgery is usually necessary.

Ankylosing Spondylitis

Ankylosing spondylitis, also known as Marie-Strümpell disease or rheumatoid spondylitis, is a form of inflammatory arthritis usually characterized by initial involvement of the sacroiliac joints, later involvement of the spinal joints, and occasional involvement of the hip joints and other joints of the body. It is much less common than rheumatoid arthritis and generally involves young men in their late teens to late twenties. The close relationship between HLA-B27 and susceptibility to ankylosing spondylitis has been known since 1973.[5] Studies have shown that approximately 20 percent of family members inheriting the B27-containing haplotype will acquire ankylosing spondylitis or a related disease.[4] HLA-B27 is present in more than 90 percent of white patients and in approximately 50 percent of American blacks with the disease. The frequency in controls runs from 4 to 8 percent.

Many people with ankylosing spondylitis remain undiagnosed, as the symptoms can be extremely mild with only minimal early morning stiffness and discomfort. The earliest radiographic findings usually involve the sacroiliac joints. Involvement of the hip joint is usually manifested by typically erosive destructive changes. Most patients with ankylosing spondylitis function relatively normally despite chronic discomfort for many years. If medical management is not sufficient to control pain and progressive deformity, surgery may be necessary.

SYSTEMIC LUPUS ERYTHEMATOSUS

Systemic lupus erythematosus (SLE), a chronic inflammatory disease of unknown origin, affects many different systems. Clinical manifestations of this disease include fever, rash, polyarthralgia and arthritis, anemia, thrombocytopenia, and renal, neurologic, and cardiac abnormalities. SLE has a strong predilection for women, especially adolescents and young adults. It occurs in black women three times as often as white women and usually follows a chronic irregular course in which episodes of disease activity are interspersed with long periods of complete or near complete remission. Patients dying from this condition usually do so as a result of vascular lesions involving the kidneys, central nervous system, or other vital organs or from complicated secondary infections.

SLE is a disease of connective tissues. A common pathologic feature is the severe vasculitis marked by cellular infiltrations of small arteries. Parts of the arterial walls may become necrotic and may contain fibrinoid deposits. The finding of a wide range of autoimmune antibodies against tissue nuclear antigens in the presence of circulating immune complexes in serum from patients with SLE provides strong support for the immunologic basis of SLE.

Joint involvement is the most common manifestation of SLE. Swelling and joint pain may precede the onset of this multisystem disease for many years. Some patients have joint pain without objective evidence of arthritis. The joints most commonly involved are the proximal interphalangeal joints, knees, wrists, and metacarpophalangeal joints. The involvement is usually symmetric. An additional explanation of hip joint pain in SLE when it occurs is avascular necrosis of the hip, which usually is secondary to the ingestion of large doses of adrenal corticosteroids over a brief period. Treatment of this multiple body systems disease usually consists of aspirin, antimalarials, and adrenal corticosteroids. Regardless of whether pain and stiffness of the hip relates to the destructive changes of SLE or avascular necrosis, surgery is usually indicated if the symptoms are not adequately controlled by a medical regimen.

AVASCULAR NECROSIS OF THE FEMORAL HEAD

Avascular necrosis is a condition in which there is progressive ischemia and secondary death of osteocytes or bone cells of the femoral head, resulting in the collapsing of bone of the femoral head and the later development of degenerative arthritis. The osteoarthritic changes are secondary to irregularity of the articular surface of the femoral head.

One of the more common causes of avascular necrosis of the femoral head is the high levels of oral steroid medication used in the treatment of inflammatory arthritis and for immunosuppression after kidney or organ transplantation. The most common form of avascular necrosis is that following hip trauma such as displaced subcapital and high transcervical fractures. The traumatic type may be associated with a healing or healed fracture. It occurs in a much older patient population and may be associated with either nonunion of the femoral head or degenerative changes of the hip joint. Nontraumatic avascular necrosis primarily affects young adults and is often bilateral.

Other causes of avascular necrosis are excess alcohol consumption, connective tissue disease such as SLE, gout, Gaucher's disease, and hemoglobinopathies. A patient with one of the previously described diseases with otherwise unexplained hip pain, or with avascular necrosis of the femoral head on the contralateral side, has a high potential of having avascular necrosis.

The pain associated with avascular necrosis is usually experienced in the groin, proximal thigh, or buttock area. One commonly sees a gradual onset; however, occasionally the onset may be sudden. Usually, there is pain and limitation of motion of the hip. Often radiographic examination reveals no abnormality in its early stages. Magnetic resonance imaging will reveal this condition before any abnormality appears on routine radiographs. A typical radiograph shows a wedge-shaped area of increased density of the articular surface of the femoral head caused by ischemia and necrosis. As the condition progresses, this necrotic bone collapses and irregularity develops in the surface of the femoral head. Later during its course, degenerative arthritic changes develop, with flattening of the femoral head, narrowing of the femoral joint, the development of sclerosis of adjacent surfaces of the joint, and cyst formation in both the acetabular and femoral margins of the joint. Treatment initially consists of limiting stress on the joint and the use of a support and, in its later stages, surgery.

BURSITIS AND TENDONITIS

A bursa is a sac or saclike cavity situated in several areas about the hip in which friction may develop (Figs. 4-1 and 4-2). Bursae are composed of synovial tissue, which has many nerve endings and can become symptomatic and painful

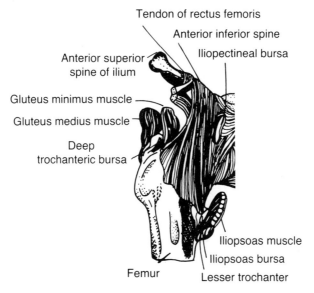

Tendon of rectus femoris
Anterior inferior spine
Iliopectineal bursa
Anterior superior spine of ilium
Gluteus minimus muscle
Gluteus medius muscle
Deep trochanteric bursa
Iliopsoas muscle
Iliopsoas bursa
Femur
Lesser trochanter

Fig. 4-1. Inflammation of the trochanteric bursa is associated with pain extending down the outer part of the thigh to the knee.

if inflammation ensues. Any bursa may be involved in a pyogenic infection, in which surgical drainage of the bursa may be necessary. The majority of symptomatic bursae showing inflammation are not associated with infectious causes and usually respond to medication.

The subgluteal bursa is large and often multiocular and is found between the gluteus maximus tendon and the greater trochanter. Inflammation of this bursa

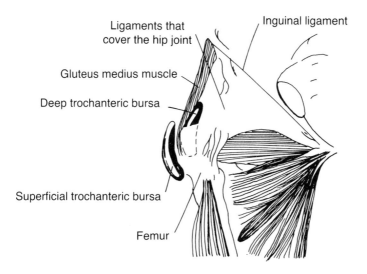

Ligaments that cover the hip joint
Inguinal ligament
Gluteus medius muscle
Deep trochanteric bursa
Superficial trochanteric bursa
Femur

Fig. 4-2. The superficial and deep bursae of the greater trochanter.

is associated with pain on the outer part of the hip in the trochanteric area and may be associated with discomfort extending down the outer part of the thigh to the knee.

The trochanteric bursa is found between the gluteus maximus tendon and the vastus lateralis muscle. Inflammation of this bursa is also associated with pain on the outer part of the thigh extending down the lateral aspect of the leg to the knee (Fig. 4-1).

The ischiogluteal bursa is adjacent to the tuberosity to the ischia. It usually becomes painful with prolonged sitting and is associated with pain in the area of the tuberosity of the ischium, which is that part of the pelvic bone that receives pressure while sitting.

The iliopsoas bursa is found between the iliopsoas tendon and lesser trochanter (Fig. 4-1). Iliopsoas bursitis can cause severe pain in the lower abdomen, groin, or upper thigh and is exacerbated by any movement of the hip joint. Ambulation can be acutely painful. A differential diagnosis may include conditions of the lower abdominal wall, such as an inguinal hernia, a pyogenic infection of the hip, an undiagnosed fracture or tumor of the proximal femur, and involvement of other bursae of the hip.

The iliopectineal bursa is found between the iliopsoas tendon and the iliopectineal eminence of the anterior pelvis (Fig. 4-1). It is associated also with lower abdominal, groin, or upper thigh pain. This bursa may communicate with the hip joint, and treatment of a pyogenic infection of this bursa may necessitate drainage of the hip joint at the same time.

Patients also can develop lateral thigh pain at or above the level of the greater trochanter from tendonitis of the abductor tendons of the hip. A radiograph of the hip region may show calcification just above the greater tuberosity involving the tendinous structures of this area. Pain from this condition usually is most severe in the area of the tip of the greater trochanter, but may appear to be coming from above this area or posterior to this area in the mid-buttock area. Usually palpation will reveal tenderness that is most severe adjacent to the greater trochanter. As with bursae of the hip, when injectable corticosteroids are used, it is very important to place the medication in the area of maximal inflammation rather than in the area that appears symptomatic to the patient. Usually heat, rest, and oral anti-inflammatory medication eliminate the patient's symptoms. Injectable corticosteroids are used if oral anti-inflammatories are not successful in eliminating pain.

SYNOVITIS

The hip joint is enclosed by a synovial membrane lying inside the ligamentous support of the hip. This synovial membrane has a rich supply of nerve endings and when inflamed can cause the hip joint to become painful. If the inflammation persists, fluid develops in the joint and further increases pain on movement of the joint. Although this condition is usually associated with degenerative changes involving the joint, it can exist as a primary condition.

Clinically, the patient complains of pain in the medial or anterolateral aspect of the hip region. The pain is increased on motion of the hip, especially in internal rotation.

Septic arthritis of the hip is found more commonly in children and is a much more serious disease in that age group. Diagnosis is made by aspiration of joint fluid. A culture and sensitivity study of the fluid reveals the organism and the appropriate antibiotic treatment. At times pus cannot be aspirated, and surgical exploration of the joint may be necessary if local and systemic symptoms cannot be otherwise explained or controlled.

OSTEOPOROSIS

Osteoporosis is a condition in which there is thinning or atrophy of bone. The most widespread metabolic bone disease, it can be associated with advanced age, immobilization, malnutrition, or endocrine disorders such as Cushing's syndrome, corticosteroid therapy, hyperthyroidism, and ovarian dysgenesis. The most common form, idiopathic osteoporosis, is seen most commonly in white women. It is often seen in patients who have had complete hysterectomies with the removal of the ovaries before the time of menopause. Senile osteoporosis usually occurs 10 years after menopause and can also be recognized in some 20 percent of men over the age of 65. The lower vertebral bodies are usually involved, and back pain is the predominant symptom.

The patient usually does not have symptoms from the hip region. When osteoporosis exists, there is usually thinning of bone in the femoral head and neck area, and most fractures of the femoral neck in the aged are associated with osteoporotic changes. Osteoporosis certainly predisposes the person to a hip fracture if trauma occurs in the region of the hip. This probably partially explains most fractures that appear to occur with twisting, stressful movements of the hip, causing fractures before the patient actually strikes the floor.

Placing normal stress on the skeleton through exercise has proved to be beneficial in maintaining good bone structure. Hormonal therapy, including estrogen and progesterone, has proved helpful in maintaining strong bone in women.

SOFT TISSUE INJURIES IN THE HIP REGION

The symptoms of injuries in the hip region can be poorly defined, and a diagnosis of the specific injury may not be easy. Injuries to the groin may mimic injuries to the hip joint, suggesting an intra-articular etiology. Pain in the groin can be caused by inflammation from overuse of a specific structure such as a muscle, tendon, or tendon attachment. Inflammatory changes associated with a tendon injury are usually thought to be due to microscopic ruptures that lead to minor tissue damage and, at times, a secondary inflammatory reaction. This symptom complex following overactivity is referred to as an overuse symptom.

Pain in the groin can also result from partial or total rupture of muscles or tendons in this area. Structures giving discomfort in the hip region upon injury include the adductor longus muscle in the groin and the lower rectus femoris and the rectus abdominis muscles in the lower abdominal area.

The muscles that draw the leg inward toward the midline in the groin area are the adductor magnus, adductor longus, adductor brevis, and pectineus muscle. The adductor longus (Fig. 4-3), the muscle most commonly injured in sports, originates from the pubic bone. Overuse of this structure can be seen in sideways kicks in soccer, track, training, and, occasionally, skating.

The pain is usually in the most proximal part of the groin, usually near the origin of the adductor longus from the pelvis. The patient may not define the pain exactly in this area; however, when the groin is examined, there is tenderness to palpation either over the area of the tear of the muscle or on the tendinous origin near the pelvic bone. There is usually an increase in pain when the leg is abducted. There may be a limp and definite decreased functional activity with sports. Occasionally, a radiograph at a later time will show calcification around the origin of the muscle from the pubic bone. Healing is seen with time and is accelerated if stress on this area is decreased.

The iliopsoas muscle is the strongest flexor of the hip joint. It inserts into the proximal portion of the femur in the area of the lesser trochanter. Inflammation of this tendon or its adjacent bursa can be seen in strength training with

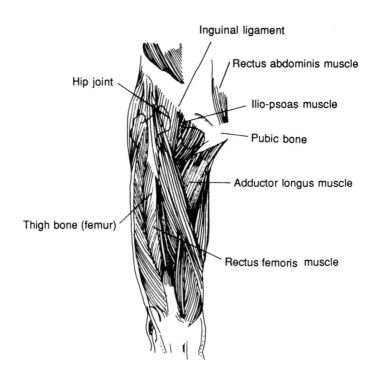

Inguinal ligament

Rectus abdominis muscle

Hip joint

Ilio-psoas muscle

Pubic bone

Adductor longus muscle

Thigh bone (femur)

Rectus femoris muscle

Fig. 4-3. Diagram of some of the muscles in the groin region.

weights, as well as with sit-ups, running uphill, and long and high jumping. It can also be seen with hurdling. The signs and symptoms from this structure can be diffuse and poorly defined. The pain can extend into the lower abdominal area as well as down along the inner aspect of the thigh. The patient's major complaint may be difficulty in putting weight on the leg and moving the leg with ambulation.

A careful examination usually will show marked tenderness to palpation in the area of the injury or the area of inflammation. Healing and disappearance of the symptoms usually follows rest and appropriate treatment.

Inflammation of the proximal portion of the rectus femoris muscle elicits pain in the region of the hip joint because of this muscle's partial origin from the anterior rim of the acetabulum. Sports involving fast starts, strength training, and repeated stressful activities of the hip joint can cause symptoms from this structure. The origin of this muscle can be involved in a rupture which, on rare occasions, is complete. It may be associated with tackling in football. Pain is usually localized to the area of the injury. Complete recovery is usually seen; however, surgery may be necessary when a complete rupture of the origin of this muscle occurs.

Inflammation or injury of the lower abdominal muscles also causes discomfort in the thigh and groin. The rectus abdominis muscle is the most common muscle involved in an injury; however, the oblique and transverse muscles of the abdomen also can be involved. Injuries, when present, are usually seen in weight lifters, throwers, rowers, wrestlers, and gymnasts. Inflammation is seen in an even wider range of sporting activities. Complete recovery is usually seen with the passage of time, a decrease in activity level, and appropriate treatment.

FRACTURES

Fractures of the proximal femur account for a higher than expected percentage of hospitalizations for the elderly and are associated with considerable morbidity and mortality. Approximately 15 to 20 percent of patients die as a direct or indirect result of these fractures. Fractures of the proximal femur are more commonly seen in women and are usually associated with osteoporosis in those over age 65. They are classified according to their anatomic location.

Fractures of the Hip

Avulsion fractures of the greater and lesser trochanter usually occur in persons under age 65 and usually do not require surgery (Fig. 4-4). Fractures between the intertrochanteric line and the base of the femoral head occur usually after a fall, although a fracture may occasionally follow a twisting movement of the hip and occur before the person strikes the floor (Fig. 4-5).

If the fracture is impacted and the superolateral aspect of the fracture site is compressed, the fracture can be treated with non-weightbearing until healing

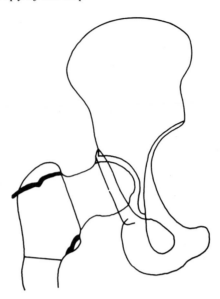

Fig. 4-4. Avulsion fracture.

occurs. If there is any question whether the patient is going to abstain from weightbearing, threaded pins are generally used for fixation, which decreases the chance of having the fracture displace. These fractures generally require 8 to 10 weeks before weightbearing can be initiated and 3 to 4 months before full weightbearing can be started.

During the immediate postfracture period, range of motion exercises should not be done as this may increase the tendency for the fracture to displace. If the fracture displaces, surgery is usually necessary. Because of the pull of the pelvic femoral muscles, nondisplaced fractures often subsequently displace and require surgery. In those over age 65, the orthopaedist will usually carry out a hemireplacement of the femoral head and neck using a femoral component such as a Thompson or Austin Moore femoral head replacement or perform a bipolar-type replacement.

There may be advantages in using a bipolar-type proximal femoral component in which there is movement between the larger portion of the prosthesis fitting into the acetabulum and the smaller prosthetic femoral head, which is directly attached to the stem and held by the proximal femur. A hemireplacement of the femoral head and neck allows earlier weightbearing; however, care must be taken to prevent a dislocation of the prosthesis. These hip prosthetic components are placed into the femoral shaft after removal of the femoral head and neck, usually through a posterior approach. Care must be taken not to allow the patient to adduct the leg or bring the leg into marked flexion, as this may dislocate the acetabular component of the prosthesis through the surgical defect in the posterior and superior capsule.

The prosthesis can also be inserted anteriorly, which may have the advantage of being associated with a smaller incidence of infection. There may also be an advantage in not creating a defect posteriorly that can allow the prosthesis to dislocate if the patient brings the hip into flexion. This is more commonly seen in the elderly senile group in which the patient may lie part of the day in bed with the hip and knee markedly flexed.

In patients under the age of 65, multiple threaded pins are usually applied across the fracture site in the femoral neck after reduction of the fracture. This procedure has the advantage of offering the patient a normal joint, assuming that the fracture heals and the circulation does not become deficient in the femoral head. The disadvantage of this procedure is that healing of the fracture site may require 3 to 6 months and may be associated with a lack of healing of the fracture site or a loss of circulation to the femoral head. The incidence of these complications may run as high as 20 to 35 percent in patients with fractures of this type. Weightbearing is safer if delayed until the patient begins to show some evidence of healing of the fracture site.

Types of Intertrochanteric Fractures

Intertrochanteric fractures are classified according to the number of parts, which is determined by the number of fracture lines (Fig. 4-5). These fractures are considered two-, three-, or four-part intertrochanteric fractures. All trochanteric fractures require surgery because of the pull of the pelvic femoral muscles. If these fractures are not treated surgically, the segments displace and the fracture goes into a varus position, causing shortening of the involved extremity. The fracture may also develop a nonunion.

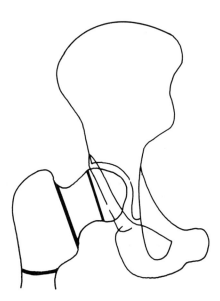

Fig. 4-5.   Intertrochanteric fracture.

Treatment includes reduction of the fracture site to restore normal anatomy and fixation, which is usually done with a compression screw for the femoral neck and head and plate that is held to the proximal femur with screws. These fractures may be classified as stable or unstable fractures. If there is continuity of bone extending from the inner portion of the femoral head down the femoral neck into the subtrochanteric area with no comminution of this area, the fracture is considered a stable one and partial weightbearing can be started earlier. This allows the patient to ambulate with a walker with less risk of displacement of the fracture site.

Unfortunately, most intertrochanteric fractures have sufficient comminution so that there is no stable column along the inner part of the proximal femoral neck and intertrochanteric areas. Because of a lack of stability, weightbearing can cause the nail to bend, break, or cut out the superior portion of the head.

Patients with unstable fractures are more safely treated with non-weightbearing, which in older patients means very limited ambulation. Toe touch gait, thought by some to limit sufficiently weightbearing on the affected extremity, usually allows the patient, especially when the fracture becomes less symptomatic, to increase weight on the leg, which increases the incidence of complications of the nailing. When initial stability is sufficient or fracture healing reaches the point at which there is enough stability for partial weightbearing, patients are started on limited ambulation using a walker. Older patients usually feel very insecure using crutches, and therefore for them a walker is the safer form of assistance for ambulation. Any patient who is secure with crutches can utilize a swing-through gait so that ambulation can be started earlier with non-weightbearing on the involved side.

Patients with an avascular necrosis of the femoral head or a nonunion after a femoral neck fracture usually require a hemi or total hip replacement, depending on the status of the articular surface of the acetabulum and the patient's age. Almost all intertrochanteric fractures heal. If the fracture does not heal, the most common reconstructive procedure performed is a hip replacement, utilizing a special femoral component to compensate for the loss of bone at the base of the femoral neck and at the level of the lesser trochanteric area.

Fractures of the Acetabulum and Dislocations of the Hip

Fractures of the acetabulum may or may not be associated with a dislocation of the hip. Dislocations of the hip are classified according to the abnormal position of the displaced femoral head and can be described as anterior, posterior, or central dislocations. Central fracture-dislocations are usually classified according to the degree of comminution and status of the weightbearing portion of the acetabulum (Fig. 4-6).

Carnesale et al.[6] have described three types of central fracture-dislocations of the hip and acetabular disruptions (Fig. 4-6).

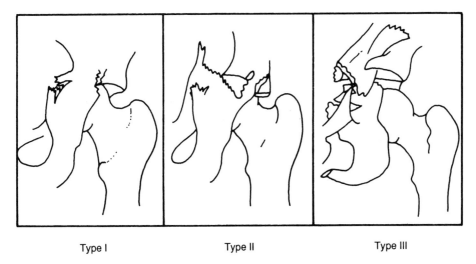

Type I   Type II   Type III

Fig. 4-6. Classification of central acetabular fractures and acetabular disruption.

Type I, or central fracture-dislocations, do not involve the weightbearing dome of the acetabulum.

Type II is a fracture involving the weightbearing dome with a central dislocation of the femoral head.

Type III is an acetabular disruption often with posterior subluxation of the hip.

The treatment of most acetabular fractures until recently involved an attempted reduction, with traction laterally and distally, and later ambulation, with no weightbearing until healing was sufficient. Traction is usually required for approximately 8 weeks, with non-weightbearing for an additional 6 to 8 weeks. With improved techniques of internal fixation, more acetabular fractures are now being treated with an open reduction with fixation consisting of screws or plates and screws.

The advantages of an open reduction are those associated with restoration of a better weightbearing surface in the acetabulum and hopefully a decreased incidence of arthritis at a later date. Even when the acetabulum cannot be perfectly reduced and secured, later reconstructive surgery consisting of a total hip replacement is easier and less likely to involve problems with good fixation at the acetabular surface of the replacement. At this time with acetabular open reductions, there is a fairly high incidence of new bone formation around the hip joint, or heterotopic bone formation, which results in stiff, symptomatic hips. This condition is currently treated with medication and low doses of radiation, which has decreased the incidence of heterotopic bone formation but has not eliminated this possibility.

Posterior dislocations of the hip are commonly associated with a fracture of the posterior portion of the acetabulum. These are classified according to the degree and location of comminution.

Thompson and Epstein[7] have classified various types of posterior dislocations of the hip with associated acetabular fractures into five groups (Fig. 4-7).

Type I consists of a posterior dislocation with or without minor fractures.

Type II is a posterior dislocation with a large simple fracture of the posterior acetabular wall.

Type III consists of a posterior dislocation with comminution of the rim of the acetabulum with or without a major fragment.

Type IV is a posterior dislocation with a fracture of the acetabular rim and floor.

Type V is a posterior dislocation with a fracture of the femoral head.

Treatment of these injuries consists of a reduction of the dislocation as soon after the injury as possible, preferably within the first 12 hours after the injury, with radiographic verification that no fracture fragments are in the joint. If the fractured segment of the posterior wall is large, the hip will be unstable in flexion, and this may be associated with a recurrent dislocation of the hip.

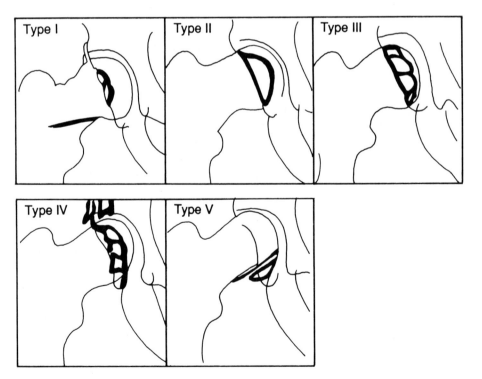

Fig. 4-7. Classification of posterior dislocations of the hip. The dislocation has been reduced.

Surgery in this case consists of reduction of the dislocation and fracture and fixation of the fractured segment with one or more screws. If one suspects a loose segment of bone in the hip joint, laminographs of the hip or a computed tomographic scan reveals the location of the entrapped fragments. Removal of the fractured fragments is necessary to prevent damage to the joint surfaces. Traction may be necessary postoperatively until sufficient healing of the posterior wall allows safe flexion without fear of dislocation of the hip. This time varies from 2 to 6 or more weeks. Patients generally progress from nonweightbearing to full weightbearing ambulation as healing occurs. Weightbearing usually is allowed when fracture healing has occurred, at approximately 12 weeks postinjury.

REFERENCES

1. Grazier KL, Holbrook TL, Kelsey JL, Stauffer RN: The frequency of occurrence, impact, and cost of musculoskeletal conditioning in the United States. The American Academy of Orthopedic Surgery, Chicago, 1984
2. Cunning LS, Kelsey JL: Epidemiology of musculoskeletal impairment and associated disability. Am J Pub Health 74:514, 579, 1984
3. Peyron JG: The epidemiology of osteoarthritis. p. 9. In Moskowitz RW, Howell DS, Goldberg VM, Mankin HG (eds): Osteoarthritis: Diagnosis and Management. WB Saunders, Philadelphia, 1984
4. Woodrow JC: Genetics and B27 associated diseases. Am Rheum Dis, suppl., 38:135–141, 1979
5. Brewerton DA, Caffrey M, Hart FD: Ankylosing spondylitis and HLA27. Lancet 1:904, 1983
6. Carnesale PG, Stewart MG, Barnes SN: Acetabular disruption and central fracture-dislocation of the hip: A long term study. J Bone Joint Surg 57A:1054, 1975
7. Thompson VP, Epstein HC: Traumatic dislocation of the hip, a survey of 204 cases covering a period of 21 years. J Bone Joint Surg 33A:746, 1951

5 | Medical and Surgical Management of the Arthritic Hip

Louis R. Jordan

Degenerative arthritis of the hip is a relatively common problem. The cause of degenerative arthritis is varied and can be divided into two main categories, primary and secondary. The primary type is also known as osteoarthritis or hypertrophic arthritis. The secondary type is secondary to some underlying etiology. This category can be classified as

1. Congenital and developmental (congenital dysplasia of the hip, Legg-Calvé-Perthes disease, slipped capital femoral epiphysis)
2. Inflammatory (rheumatoid arthritis, juvenile rheumatoid arthritis, ankylosing spondylitis)
3. Traumatic (fractures of the acetabulum or femoral head or neck, dislocation of a hip)
4. Avascular necrosis
5. Tumors (malignant and nonmalignant)
6. Metabolic
7. Hereditary
8. Failed previous hip reconstruction
9. Infection

With the longevity of today's population increasing, the elderly population will become more numerous and, correspondingly, arthritic problems, both primary and secondary, will become more prevalent. As a result, not only will there be

69

the usual number of younger and middle-aged patients with degenerative arthritis, there will be an even larger number of elderly people with degenerative arthritis of the hip.

The medical and surgical treatment of arthritis of the hip has evolved over the years to the point that today the majority of patients with a painful, arthritic hip can be relieved of this pain and returned to a more normal quality of life.

MEDICAL MANAGEMENT

Initially, the etiology of the painful, arthritic hip should be determined. Once this has been accomplished, the patient should be treated conservatively according to the etiology of the hip disease. If, after an adequate trial of conservative management, the patient continues to have pain, loss of function, and a decrease in the quality of life, surgical intervention remains a viable option.

The medical management of a painful, arthritic hip varies somewhat according to the etiology of the hip disease. For any patient with persistent hip pain, a complete medical evaluation is essential before any treatment is instituted. This evaluation should include medical history, physical examination, and appropriate diagnostic tests.

The medical history should include questions related to birth or childhood hip problems, previous illnesses, medications, operations, allergies, and accidents. It should include questions regarding localization of the pain. Most hip pain is related to the groin area, greater trochanter, anterior thigh, and occasionally the knee. It is also important to know when the pain bothers the patient. Does it hurt on walking, standing, going up and down stairs, getting out of a sitting position, sitting, or lying in bed at night? Has the patient had any functional loss such as limitation of motion of the hip, difficulty putting on shoes and stockings, getting out of a bathtub, squatting, kneeling, or crossing the legs? Last, it is important to make sure that the pain is not being referred from some other area such as the back.

The physical examination should include watching the patient walk, sit, and go up and down stairs. The range of motion of both hips, pelvic tilt, leg length discrepancies, and muscle strength should be noted, and the neuromuscular status of the leg should be evaluated. A similar evaluation should be done on the opposite extremity whether or not it is symptomatic.

The back, knees, ankles, and feet should be evaluated for any deformities or loss of motion. Finally, the upper extremities should be examined for function and strength since crutches or a walker will be needed in the immediate postoperative period. Patients with rheumatoid arthritis may have upper extremity involvement requiring modifications of walkers or crutches so that they may ambulate in the postoperative period without much difficulty.

Diagnostic testing is important to complete the patient's evaluation. This includes roentgenograms of both hips and the femoral shaft of the involved hip. Occasionally, more sophisticated studies such as the bone scan, magnetic resonance imaging, computed tomography, or arthrograms are needed to delineate further the patient's hip problem. Other important laboratory tests include a complete blood count, urinalysis, erythrocyte sedimentation rate, blood sugar, uric acid, and rheumatoid factor.

Once the cause of the arthritic hip pain has been determined, appropriate treatment can be instituted. Except perhaps for tumorous conditions, the initial treatment is conservative or nonoperative. Benign tumors can be treated, if necessary, by resection and primary reconstruction. Malignant tumors, depending on the pathologic type and the degree of malignancy, can also be treated by resection and reconstruction of the hip.

In general, degenerative arthritis of the hip, whether it is primary or secondary, is initially treated by conservative measures. Many times this conservative regimen will prolong the life of the hip for many years, thus avoiding or delaying surgical intervention. Conservative measures include instructing the patient on the care of the hip and helping the patient understand the mechanics of the hip, the magnitude of stresses that are placed across the hip joint, and how the patient can help maintain the integrity of hip function. The patient must understand the role that rest, medication and change in life style play in prolonging the life of the arthritic hip joint. It is of extreme importance to decrease the stresses and decrease the inflammation of the hip joint to accomplish this goal.

Decreasing the stress is accomplished by unloading the hip as much as possible. This can be done by appropriate muscle-strengthening exercises. Increasing the strength of the hip musculature not only helps reduce the stress on the hip preoperatively but enables the patient to recover postoperatively in a more timely manner. Muscle rehabilitation and strengthening can be done through weight lifting, bicycling, and swimming. One should avoid high-impact activities such as running, jogging, tennis, racquetball, and even unnecessary walking or stair climbing. These activities greatly increase the stresses across the hip joint. When walking in the stance phase of gait, the forces across the hip joint are three times the body weight. When running or jumping, the load may be ten times the body weight.[1] These stresses in cyclic loading occur over a million times a year, so anything that can be done to decrease the amount of cyclic loading activity will help to prolong the function of the hip. One can consider an arthritic hip in its early stages before surgery as a ball bearing beginning to wear out. The more one uses it, the quicker it will deteriorate. The more one protects it, the longer it will last. In regard to exercise, one should not forget to keep the upper extremities in good condition because eventually, if surgery is done, postoperatively external support in the form of crutches or a walker will be needed for a time. Another way to decrease the load on the hip is by using a cane in the opposite hand or crutches or a walker. The weightbearing should be partial since this unloads the hip more than complete non-weightbearing.[2] Last, weight reduction will decrease the forces across the hip joint and is essential in any preoperative and postoperative management of arthritis of the hip.

Further relief of stress of the hip can be provided by bed rest or even a wheelchair. Short periods of rest during the day are helpful but should be tempered with the realization that excessive bed rest or use of a wheelchair can lead to weakening musculature, atrophy, joint contractures, and osteoporosis.

Inflammation and pain of the joint can be decreased not only by rest, limited weightbearing, and heat but also by the use of anti-inflammatory medication. This can be in the form of aspirin, nonsteroidal anti-inflammatory drugs, and occasionally locally injected or oral corticosteroids. Analgesics can also be used during periods of acute pain but, like any habit-forming medication, should be used cautiously in long-term treatment.

There are some situations in which treatment is more specific, such as rheumatoid arthritis or gout. Rheumatoid arthritis is frequently treated with gold injections, systemic corticosteroids, aspirin, or nonsteroidal anti-inflammatory drugs. Gout is treated with uricosuric drugs to avoid the gouty inflammatory arthritis.

If symptoms and disability persist despite the conservative measures, and the patient's quality of life is deteriorating, then surgical intervention can be considered. Patients, however, should be fairly appraised of the indications, alternatives, complications, consequences thereof, and expectations. They should realize that, although surgical intervention gives them an excellent chance of improvement, they will never have a completely normal hip, and certain limitations will be placed on them postoperatively.

SURGICAL MANAGEMENT

Although total hip replacement is the most common operative procedure for degenerative hip disease, other procedures are available. Since one of the concerns of total hip replacement is longevity of the prosthesis and its fixation, these procedures can be used to gain time until the patient gets older.

Intertrochanteric osteotomy can be used to relieve the pain of arthritis. In this procedure, the femur is cut at the intertrochanteric level and the neck shaft angle is changed or rotated to allow more healthy articulating cartilage to become involved in the weightbearing stresses. The osteotomy also may alter the vascularity to the femoral head, and this may influence the progression of symptoms of osteoarthritis. Finally, the osteotomy affects the forces exerted by the various muscles about the hip and, in turn, helps in the relief of pain. The exact mechanism of pain relief, however, is unknown but most likely is due, as mentioned, to change in the stress and weight transfer across the hip joint both passively and actively. The long-term results, however, are somewhat unpredictable as to relief of pain, and today this is thought to be a temporizing procedure reserved for younger patients in whom temporary pain relief is desired. This allows the patient to lead a more unrestricted life style for an additional 5 or 10 years until the age is reached when a total joint reconstruction would be more realistic.

Arthrodesis or fusion of the hip is an excellent procedure for relief of pain. This is indicated in the younger, vigorous patient, especially the active man involved in manual labor with unilateral hip disease. These patients must be willing to accept a stable but stiff hip in exchange for relief of pain. Once the hip is fused, the patient usually will not need any further hip surgery, although it is possible at a later date to revise this to a total hip arthroplasty. It is not indicated for patients with arthritis of the lower back, and it is less desirable if the patient has severe arthritis of the opposite hip or ipsilateral knee. It is also less desirable if the patient's occupation is more sedentary.

Prosthetic replacement of the arthritic femoral head in osteoarthritis of the hip is usually not indicated unless the degeneration is limited to the femoral head. Since the prosthesis only replaces the femoral side of the hip joint, if the acetabular side is also involved with arthritic changes, this procedure will eventually have to be converted to a total hip reconstruction. Femoral head prosthetic replacement (bipolar hip) is reserved for avascular necrosis of the femoral head, fractures of the femoral neck, or tumors of the proximal femur. Occasionally in cases of severe acetabular deficiency, the bipolar prosthesis in association with bone grafting has been used to help reconstruct acetabular defects.

In general, given the proper indication, the total hip prosthesis is the procedure of choice for the surgical treatment of degenerative arthritis of the hip. Over 150,000 total hip replacements are done yearly, and as longevity increases and the elderly population increases, the number will continue to grow.[2] The goals of the surgery are mainly to relieve pain and improve function, range of motion, and ambulatory capacity and to enable the patient to achieve a more normal life style. Initially, total hip replacements were indicated for those patients 65 years or older, but as experience has accumulated and the designs and methods of fixation have improved, the age limit has been lowered to include the younger patient.

If a patient has had an intensive trial of conservative management, has lost or tried to lose weight, has tried external support, anti-inflammatory medications, and exercise programs with restricted activity, and despite these measures has pain at night and pain on motion, standing, walking, and stair climbing sufficient to interfere with work or activities of daily living, then the patient is a candidate for total hip reconstruction. This is provided there are no contraindications to surgery.

Contraindications to total hip surgery include active infection either in the hip joint or elsewhere in the body, skeletally immature individuals, and those patients with a neurotrophic joint, progressive neurologic disease, or who are unlikely to walk after surgery. Patients should also have sufficient bone stock available into which to insert the total hip prosthesis, and thus the quality and quantity of bone around the hip should be evaluated preoperatively. Various medical problems (cardiovascular, pulmonary, genitourinary, gastrointestinal, metabolic, or neurologic) may contraindicate surgery; total hip replacement patients should be evaluated preoperatively for any of these problems.

Complications, although rare (1 to 2 percent), should be discussed with the patient preoperatively. Infection is one of the most devastating complications since its occurrence can negate an otherwise excellently performed total hip reconstruction. For this reason, the body should be cleared preoperatively of any infection. Also, there should be strict adherence to sterile technique during surgery, and preoperative, intraoperative, and postoperative broad-spectrum antibiotic coverage should be used.

The main intraoperative complications include fractures of the femur or acetabulum, injuries to the nerves or blood vessels surrounding the hip, significant blood loss, reactions to general anesthesia, and hypotension secondary to fat embolization.

Postoperatively, the more serious early complications are dislocation of the hip, infections, venous thrombosis, and pulmonary emboli. Late complications include infections, component loosening, and occasionally dislocation or fracture of the femur after a traumatic episode.

A total joint prosthesis as it is known today is made up of an acetabular and a femoral component. There are many designs of total hip components, but most acetabular components are a combination of a metal shell with an ultra-high-molecular-weight polyethylene articulating inner surface. The femoral component has a chrome-cobalt head and a stem frequently made of titanium alloy. The chrome-cobalt head has superior wear for the articulating surface, and the titanium alloy stem is excellent for stress transfer. The acetabular cups and femoral stems come in a variety of sizes to better match the patient's own bony anatomy.

One of the primary problems in total hip replacements is to ensure a painless long-term fixation of the prosthesis.[3] Today the components are fixed to the bone either with polymethyl methacrylate cement or by bone ingrowth into a roughened porous surface on the implant. Other prosthetic designs have femoral components with grooves to help give a tight fit when the component is press fitted into the femoral canal. The porous surface either is made of a fine titanium wire mesh or is formed by sintering small beads of metal onto the surface of the implant. Bone grows into these porous surfaces and thus stabilizes the components to the bone.

Long-term aseptic loosening of cemented total hip replacements has been a problem, especially in younger, more active patients. Chandler et al.[4] noted 57 percent actual or pending loosening at 5 years postoperatively in patients under 30 years of age. Dorr et al.[5] noted 45 percent impending failures at 4.5 years in patients under 45 years of age, and Amstutz et al.[6] noted failure rates of 10.6 percent at 5 years in patients under 55 years old. In patients 40 years old and younger, the estimated rate for aseptic loosening was 30.3 percent; in patients 40 to 65 years, it was 7.0 percent; and in patients older than 65 years, it was 5.5 percent.[6] Thus, proper patient selection is important because evidence supports an increased failure rate with increased weight, younger age, and higher activity level.

Because of this problem of potential loosening with time, attention has been directed to the use of noncemented implants, especially in the younger age group. Fixation of these components relies on bone ingrowth, and although early results are encouraging as to fixation of the components, long-term follow-up is still lacking. Bone ingrowth, like fracture healing, is somewhat unpredictable. Therefore, it is still somewhat premature to say that cementless fixation is the ultimate method of fixation. Although one can find any combination of cement or cementless fixation, cementing one or both of the components, or cementing neither, there is a tendency for most patients to receive a noncemented acetabular component. This noncemented component is press fitted into the bony acetabulum and is fixed to the acetabular bone by screws drilled through the holes in a metal cup into the acetabular bone or by small spikes or by pegs that are press fitted into the bony acetabulum. In younger patients, a noncemented femoral component is frequently used; in those patients over 60 years of age, the femoral component is usually, but not always, cemented. In revision total hip reconstruction (reoperations for previous failed total hip procedures), the noncemented prosthesis along with appropriate bone grafting is usually employed.

Postoperative Management

Postoperatively, the management is the same whether or not cement is used. The exception is the weightbearing status. Both the noncemented and the cemented total hip replacement patients are allowed out of bed the day after surgery. Both are started on quadriceps, abduction, and straight-leg-raising exercising. They are taught to avoid those positions that might cause dislocation of the hip, namely, flexion beyond 90°, internal rotation beyond 0°, and adduction beyond 0°. They are therefore advised to use elevated seats, avoid soft chairs, avoid squatting, avoid crossing their legs, and avoid sleeping on the unoperated side (this has a tendency to cause the operated leg to go into adduction and internal rotation, thus possibly leading to dislocation) until the fibrous capsule heals. This usually takes approximately 3 to 4 months.

The patient with a cemented total hip replacement can bear weight as tolerated with crutches the day after surgery and can progress to a cane and eventually no support as confidence is gained, strength returns, and pain subsides. The patient with a noncemented hip replacement should have partial weightbearing (toe touch) for a minimum of 6 weeks. The success of the cementless prosthesis depends on the bone ingrowth. Bone ingrowth is inhibited by any motion, even micromotion, at the bone-prosthetic interface, and it takes approximately 6 weeks for the bone to incorporate into the fiber mesh or porous surface. For the next 6 weeks, the patient is allowed to use a cane for protected weightbearing to allow the ingrown bone to become more mature. At the end of 3 months, both types of patients are allowed to resume more normal daily activities. They may return to such activities as bowling, swimming, bicycling, and golf but are discouraged from participating in high-impact sports or activities such as running, tennis, racquetball, and skiing. By avoiding these high-impact activities, it is hoped that loosening will be prevented and the longevity of the components will be prolonged.

FUTURE CONSIDERATIONS

Research is being done on improving methods of fixation (hydroxyapatite tricalcium phosphate, porous polymers), newer alloys are being developed, and ways to develop better-fitting implants are being explored. Materials such as ceramics are being evaluated for use on the femoral or acetabular side since they appear to have excellent wear qualities and are well tolerated by the body. Finally, the use of human allografts to replace the entire joint is being considered and may be still another solution for the painful arthritic joint. The goal of the future is to produce a total hip prosthesis that will not loosen, that will wear indefinitely, and that will last the lifetime of the patient. With continued research and the development of new materials and fixation methods, this should become a reality.

REFERENCES

1. Callanndruccio RA: Arthroplasty of hip. p. 1213. In Crenshaw AH (ed): Campbell's Operative Orthopaedics. 7th Ed. Vol. 2. CV Mosby, St. Louis, 1987
2. Kozinn SC, Wilson PD, Jr: Adult disease and total hip replacement. Clinical Symposia 39, 1987
3. Mayor MB: Symposium: Bony ingrowth of prosthesis (cemented or uncemented). Contemp Orthop 14:81, 1987
4. Chandler HP, Reineck FT, Wixson RL, et al: Total hip replacement in patients younger than thirty years old. J Bone Joint Surg 63A:1426, 1981
5. Dorr LD, Take GK, Conaty JB: Total hip arthroplasties in patients less than forty-five years old. J Bone Joint Surg 65A:474, 1983
6. Amstutz HC, Yao J, Dorey FJ, et al: Survival analysis of T-29 hip arthroplasty with clinical implications. Orthop Clin North Am 19:491, 1981

6 | Rehabilitation of Total Hip Replacements and Fracture Management Considerations

George C. Maihafer

From the beginning, physical therapists have played a crucial role in the rehabilitation of patients with orthopaedic conditions requiring total hip replacement (THR). The nature of our profession places the therapist in the position of being an evaluator, health care provider, and educator to these patients throughout all phases of their hospital stay and rehabilitation experiences. Historically, physical therapists have worked closely with orthopaedic surgeons on the rehabilitative aspects of fracture management. It has been documented that patients who receive rehabilitation from a skilled professional achieve greater independence and control over their lives in a shorter time than those patients who are left to their own devices postoperatively.[1,2] It should therefore not be surprising that the physical therapist is viewed as a valued and essential member of the rehabilitation team in THR patient care when these factors are taken into consideration. Therapists working in acute care settings had enhanced the quality of life and efficiency of recovery in postsurgical orthopaedic patients long before the advent of joint replacement surgery. Our role in preoperative instruction, evaluation, and postoperative care of THR patients is a logical step from the past contributions provided to these patients.

In recent years, the financial constraints placed on patients and hospitals in the form of medical insurance premiums and reimbursement policies, respectively, have added a greater urgency toward improving the efficiency and time spent in the rehabilitation of THR patients. Health care delivery is recognized as a business, and patient outcome is its product. The health care industry measures success not only in terms of the quality of life achieved but also by the efficiency with which these results were obtained. More than ever before, physical therapists are being asked to review their protocols, set measurable standards for patient success, and improve the efficiency of their rehabilitation approaches for THR patients.[3] Physical therapy, because of its critical role in rehabilitation care, is recognized as an important element in achieving these goals to the satisfaction of everyone concerned in the patient's well-being. To better understand the rehabilitation protocols and goals currently in use for THR patients, a review of the development of artificial implant designs as an approach in treating diseases and trauma to the hip joint may be useful.

DEVELOPMENT OF TOTAL HIP REPLACEMENTS

Total joint replacement surgery is a common procedure performed in many acute care hospitals today. THR procedures are a relatively recent surgical phenomenon in this country, however, having been performed on a large scale only in the last 25 years. Cup arthroplasties of Vitallium (cobalt-chromium) alloy, designed by Smith-Petersen, were the treatment of choice for surgical intervention of degenerative joint disease of the hip from the 1930s until the mid-1960s.[4] The simplicity in design of this acetabular replacement, coupled with research documenting remarkable success rates after 15 years of follow-up studies, made this surgical replacement an obvious favorite among orthopaedic surgeons. Even today many Vitallium cup arthroplasties are reported to be successfully functioning after 30 years of wear. In recent years, Vitallium has given way to the use of polymers in acetabular cup design, such as the ultra-high-molecular-weight polyethylene used in today's cup implants. This material exhibits high wear resistance and a low coefficient of surface friction.

The development of the femoral component and the method of its surface bonding have not been as easily achieved nor met with universal acceptance among orthopaedic surgeons even today. At the turn of the century, Theophilus Gluck designed surgical hip implants using ivory. Californium, pumice, and plaster of Paris were combined to form the cementing agent. These implants suffered extrusion after several months of wear. Over the next 60 years, medical researchers continued to experiment using various materials in the design of the femoral components and cementing mixture with little long-term success. Stainless steel implants, which had the characteristic of tensile strength, tended to corrode over time, resulting in infections and rejection. Cementing agents were either too toxic or failed to hold the femoral stem in place, causing loosening, fractures, and dislocations.

Ultimately, for long-term success in artificial implants to take place, the following prerequisites must be met[5]:

Biologic compatibility
Adequate strength and wear resistance
Implants that mirror normal biomechanics as closely as possible
Implants that are not adversely affected by the biologic environment (e.g., corrosion-resistant alloys, biostable polymers)
Low friction wear between surfaces

Rehabilitation protocols involving specific exercises, activities, and weightbearing instruction would also be considered a prerequisite to the long-term success of any total joint program. In the 1960s, Charnley developed a femoral component that demonstrated successful results in 4- and 6-year clinical trials.[4] The material—casted chromium, cobalt, and molybdenum (Co-Cr-Mo)—demonstrated acceptable tensile strength while resisting corrosion and tissue rejection. Prevention of dislocation was not so much a function of design but rather of the fibrous capsule that formed around the new joint. This relative instability continues to have implications in the rehabilitation of THR patients. Implant loosening and traumatic dislocations are seen in falls or extremes of movement, particularly hip flexion, and are therefore avoided at all costs during rehabilitation. One key factor in the success of THR was Charnley's use of cold curing acrylic cement, a process that allows contact and stresses distributed between the prosthesis and the bone over a larger surface area.[4] This cementing agent, polymethyl methacrylate (PMMA), bonds the metal implant to the intra-medullary canal by forming an interlocking network between the irregularities.[6] Surgical procedures using this or any other femoral implant design emphasize the reaming of the intramedullary canal and the insertion of the PMMA under pressure to maximize the bonding between the two surfaces. Disadvantages of PMMA include relatively poor tensile and compressive strengths, with a modulus of elasticity approximately one-eighth that of cortical bone. Despite the reported success in THR procedures, a number of patients still require further revision or replacement surgery owing to implant failure or cement loosening. Nevertheless, THR procedures have represented a superior approach in the management of certain hip fractures and arthritic conditions. Before the introduction of THR surgery in the late 1960s, hip fractures were considered one of the leading causes of mortality in the elderly.[7] Conventional treatment had required a long period of immobilization in bed, often resulting in respiratory complications and death. Even today, hip fractures among the elderly are responsible for a mortality rate reported from 1.3 to 16 percent during the immediate postoperative period. Hip fracture management is also recognized as a significant financial burden to the patient and a resource drain on acute care facilities. Although discharge diagnoses in U.S. hospitals rank hip fractures at only 55th, they still rank 10th in total days spent in the hospital.[7]

Physical therapy departments quickly responded to the new patient population by developing specific protocols for postoperative rehabilitation, often under the direct guidance and supervision of the orthopaedic surgeon.

The newness of the procedure, coupled with the previously mentioned potential for implant failure, dictated a strictly regimented, conservative approach during physical rehabilitation. Preoperative instructions were commonly provided by the nursing and surgical staffs. Patients were seen bedside postoperatively by the physical therapist 2 to 3 days after surgery. Patients were brought to the department by stretcher; weightbearing was achieved through the use of the tilt table. Patients were mobilized, through ambulation and exercise, at a much earlier time in their recovery than with the previous methods of hip fracture management. An alternative treatment for severe degenerative arthritis of the hip was likewise now available. Independent ambulation with assistive devices and discharge generally occurred 10 days to 2 weeks postoperatively, substantially diminishing length of hospital stay and mortality figures.

As implant design, surgical technique, and clinical research developed through the 1970s, the rigid, conservative rehabilitation protocols were altered to reflect more diverse and progressive regimens. These were determined by the physician's experience, surgical approach, patient status, and the increasing number of varied surgical implant designs on the market. Physical therapists, whose numbers and responsibilities in acute care settings grew during the 1970s, increased their participation in planning the rehabilitation of THR patients. Clearly written protocols were developed, underscoring the therapist's role in preoperative evaluation and instruction, postoperative therapy, and functional home and work assessments for discharge planning.

The protocols presented in this chapter reflect the experience that has been developed over the years by orthopaedic surgeons and physical therapists who have worked with the rehabilitation of THR patients.

In the past 10 years, an alternative surgical approach and design fabrication has been added to the management of the total hip arthroplasty. In the early 1970s, MacNab and Campbell[8] began experimental research clinical trials using a porous coated hip prosthesis that would allow for biologic fixation without the need for a cementing agent such as PMMA. After successful clinical trials in Canada and the United States, the federal Food and Drug Administration approved for general use the porous coated total hip prosthesis. The prosthesis, which resembles a modified Austin Moore femoral component, enables biologic fixation by its design. A large number of fixation points can be achieved through bony ingrowth, thereby transmitting loads over a large surface area and minimizing the stresses placed on the bone-implant interface. Long-term stability of this bond is achieved owing to the constant bone remodeling that occurs as a result of normal stresses over time at the interface.

Regardless of the underlying theory of biologic fixation in THR, the postoperative program of rehabilitation in physical therapy is altered to reflect the rate of recovery and rehabilitation progression in this procedure. The field of orthopaedics is presently debating the pros and cons of both schools of thought in total joint replacement.[9,10] Proponents of the biologic fixation approach state that the bone-remodeling characteristic provides the THR patient with a greater chance for long-term function and stability than the cemented implant approach.[9] Clinical researchers who prefer implant fixation by cementing agent point out that adequate longitudinal studies of biologic implants have not been performed; far too many patients complain of residual long-term pain and limp. They also are not entirely convinced that bony ingrowth is actually taking place or is the method of fixation.[10] Researchers state that past failures of cemented components were due to the lack of knowledge of the biomechanical properties of PMMA. With new preparation techniques, such as high-vacuum mixing and chilling of the cement, implant failure rates of 1 percent and lower are now being reported in the literature.[11,12] In the foreseeable future, it appears that both methods of total joint replacement will be used by surgeons, depending on their medical experience, patient profiles, and professional preference. Since the two methods pose different challenges and precautions to physical therapists during the patients' recovery stages, it is necessary to understand the implications for successful rehabilitation of both surgical procedures.

CONSIDERATIONS FOR SUCCESSFUL REHABILITATION

The general goals of a successful rehabilitation program for THR patients focus on the following:

Pain-free motion of the postoperative leg
Independent ambulation, with no gait disturbance
Functional independence in activities of daily living

We know that realistically many patients will not fully achieve all these goals. Indeed, in some cases preoperative status finds the surgical candidate unable to ambulate independently or exhibit a functional range of motion. Kumar and Redford[7] report that, when working with the elderly, a hip fracture is indeed "unsolvable if medical care is directed at only treating the fracture and not the patient as a whole. A good surgical outcome requires intensive rehabilitation." The geriatric population of the United States will continue to represent a significant percentage of the overall population through 2050, owing in large part to longer life spans and the aging of the post-World War II generation.[8] It is plausible to assume this population will have its share of THR candidates and the need for physical therapy services. It is also prudent to realize that patients over the age of 65 are now more active and live longer and more productive and demanding lives than ever before.

All too often in present day practice it is my observation that some patients receive surgery without preoperative evaluation or instructions from therapists and that patients are discharged from some facilities without the knowledge of the therapist. These failures in communication undermine the potential for achieving a successful outcome for the patient. If such occurrences repeat on a regular basis, therapists and the medical staff should take steps to recognize the problems and rectify the situation. Successful outcomes in rehabilitation for THR patients can only develop when all members of the medical team are communicating and working toward a common goal.

REHABILITATION PROTOCOLS

Preoperative Evaluation and Instruction

The common theme presented in the literature on THR is that clear, concise, and reinforced instruction and careful evaluation during the preoperative stage improve the motivation, understanding, and compliance in rehabilitation of the postsurgical patient.[13] Most agree that goals should be developed with functional performance in mind, taking into consideration the patient's physical status, cognitive understanding, and level of independence. The exception to this principle is the patient's report of pain and discomfort. A THR will not be classified as successful if the patient's preoperative level of pain has not diminished or vanished after surgery.

One study investigated the importance of a well-defined, structured program of preoperative instructions to THR patients' overall understanding, attitude, and postoperative outcome.[3] The instructional package for the experimental group included written materials and verbal presentations describing the surgical procedure, immediate postoperative experiences, and expected long-term benefits of the joint replacement. A pretest, post-test, and slide-tape series were used to reinforce further the experimental group's knowledge of their hospital experience. The control group received the standard protocol of preoperative evaluation and verbal and written review of the postoperative rehabilitation program. The results found no difference in patient group performance, length of hospital stay, or level of postoperative complications. The researchers did find that the experimental group demonstrated greater recall of the rehabilitation protocol, were more compliant in therapy sessions, and reported greater satisfaction with their hospital experiences than the control group.[3] Ley and associates[14] studied the length of time and amount of recall acute care patients exhibited when information was given to them by the medical staff. The researchers found that within 5 minutes of the instructional encounter, patients forgot one-half of what they were told. Recall of knowledge was greatly enhanced when written instructions were given to patients with periodic reinforcement and cueing by the staff.

Most physical therapy departments have developed protocols for preoperative THR patient evaluation and instruction. These vary from facility to facility. They are often determined and governed by the orthopaedic surgeon's program for postoperative care and the surgical implant and procedure used. The preoperative assessment should consider the following questions:

1. What is the patient's preoperative level of pain, range of motion, and muscle strength?
2. Before this time, was the patient employed, and if so, what occupation?
3. What has been the patient's preoperative ambulatory status?
4. Is the patient independent in activities of daily living (i.e., bathing, dressing, housework)?
5. Is the patient able to get in and out of a car? Climb stairs?

Table 6-1. Preoperative Physiotherapy Evaluation: THR Patient

System/Category	Examination Procedure	Comments
Respiratory	Perform chest examination, expansion breath sounds reported	Instruct patient in postoperative breathing exercises
Gait	Evaluate gait pattern, use of ambulation aides, wearing areas on footwear	Explain postoperative precautions involving weightbearing, transfers, use of ambulation aides
Posture	Evaluate preoperative leg length discrepancy, fixed hip flexion deformity via Thomas test	Instruct patient in proper postures (i.e., avoid hip rotations, adduction extremes in flexion)
Range of motion; hip and knee strength	Perform manual muscle test and goniometric measures	Discuss postoperative exercise protocol

(Modified courtesy of R. Carter, senior physiotherapist: Austin Hospital, Heidelberg Victoria 3084, Australia, 1989.)

Table 6-1 is an example of the preoperative evaluation and instruction criteria from the physical therapy department's point of view from Austin Hospital in Australia. The surgical team of this facility commonly chooses to use the cemented Charnley prosthesis for patients over the age of 70; a porous coated implant with biologic fixation is used in those patients under 70 years of age. The biologic fixation implant is believed to withstand greater stresses from more active adults over time because of the bone ingrowth's capacity to remodel.[15] This protocol also emphasizes pulmonary evaluation and instruction in breathing exercises as an integral part of the early stages of recovery. The preoperative evaluation of the respiratory status of the patient is essential in determining a baseline by which the patient's postoperative pulmonary condition may be measured.

Information obtained on the gait pattern and musculoskeletal status of the preoperative patient provides the therapist with a baseline by which rehabilitation gain may be measured in the days and weeks to come. The therapist who is able to determine factors such as leg length discrepancies, muscle contractures, and weakness will be able to anticipate these problems in rehabilitation and plan the treatment programs accordingly. The comprehensive preoperative evaluation will consequently save time for the patient and therapist while speeding up the recovery process.

In addition to performing a preoperative evaluation, the physical therapist will instruct the THR patient in postoperative exercises, the expected stages of rehabilitation, and the precautions to specific movements and activities. Routine explanations regarding the operation, anesthesia reactions, and immediate hours after surgery are generally handled by the surgical or nursing staff. Clear communication and protocol review among all members of the rehabilitation team are necessary, so that important information is not missing or contradicted in the verbal and written instructions to the surgical candidate.

Hospital admittance for surgery is an emotionally unsettling time for patients. The elderly THR patient may appear distracted, noncompliant, or confused owing to the new surroundings and unfamiliar faces. It is essential that the information given to the patients is clear and concise, does not contradict other authorities, and is reinforced throughout the hospital stay.

Appendix 6-1 is an example of a patient instruction sheet for bed exercises, in this case utilizing slings, springs, and rolls. Appendix 6-2 is a similar selection of another protocol for THR patients, in this case not using any assistive devices for the exercise regimen. Both designed protocols represent typical THR bed exercise programs given to the patients. The exercises are clearly written, avoiding too much medical jargon, while using pictures to reinforce each command. The exercises offered at the top of each sheet are usually performed during the first few hours and days postoperatively, with more physically demanding exercises added during the recovery process.

Therapists are advised to individualize these programs by adding or subtracting exercises depending on the patient's postoperative condition. Additional preoperative instructions to the patient may address the following immediate postoperative concerns:

1. Most THR procedures require the presence of an abduction pillow or wedge placed between the legs when the patient is in bed or in a wheelchair.
2. Patients are cautioned not to exceed 90° of flexion of the operative hip.
3. Passive or forcible movement of the hip that causes pain is contraindicated.
4. Internal rotation and adduction are contraindicated.
5. The patient is encouraged to perform active ankle exercises—rhythmic active dorsal and plantar flexion—frequently during the first few days postoperatively to prevent thrombophlebitis.
6. No weightbearing or standing should take place unless under the direct supervision of the physical therapist.
7. Transfers and log rolling should be performed away from the operative side, with the leg supported by a staff member.

These instructions should also be given to the patient as written material for reinforcement. The therapist should demonstrate the activities and have the patient perform as many of the exercises as possible before surgery.

Postoperative Rehabilitation

Whereas THR patients 20 years ago started postoperative rehabilitation only after a few days of bed rest, today's patient often commences bedside physical therapy within 24 hours of the surgery.[15] The patient's physical status is assessed throughout the recovery period based on the regimen chosen for rehabilitation. The initial physical therapy focuses on pain-free active range of motion measurements and exercises on the operated side. Reviewing the proper method of changing positions in bed is also critical so that injuries such as suture tears, dislocation of the prosthesis, or femoral fractures do not occur. At this time, the need for an overhead bed trapeze and instruction in its use are indicated. In subsequent days as the patient's exercise program includes bridging and log rolling, the trapeze may be removed.

Kumar and Redford[7] report that postoperative complications commonly seen in elderly patients with hip fractures include thromboembolism, bed sores, pneumonia, and confusion owing to the anesthesia administered during surgery. Physical therapy during the first few days addresses these potential problems through active exercises, as seen in Appendices 6-1 and 6-2, and isometric strengthening programs emphasizing the quadriceps, hamstrings, and gluteal muscles. Pulmonary therapy utilizing breathing exercises and postural drainage is employed to forestall respiratory complications seen in postoperative stages. Physical therapy is recommended a minimum of twice a day, and more active exercises are added in subsequent sessions as the patient recovers. Functional independence in ambulation and activities of daily living of the THR patient are the main goals of the postoperative rehabilitation experience. Pain is an important governing factor, and no exercise or movement should increase the patient's discomfort after surgery. Normal neuromuscular performance preparatory to gait training can only take place when pain is eliminated from the activity. Reviewing the patient's preoperative status will provide the therapist with a pragmatic view of the patient's potential for functional performance and the pace at which this may be achieved.

The bedside therapy program is completed with instructions in transfer techniques. A wheelchair or stretcher will be used in transferring the THR patient to the physical therapy department exercise area depending on the mode of transportation chosen by the surgeon or the rehabilitation protocol employed. The abduction pillow should be used while transporting the patient. The patient being transported in a wheelchair should be in a semireclined position for the first week after surgery. Like the exercise programs, gait training is an individualized approach depending on the age of the patient, physical status, surgical protocol, physician's preference, etc. Table 6-2 is an example of four different gait protocols used for THR patients at Medical College of Virginia hospitals. This table illustrates a number of important facts. The trochanteric osteotomy presents the most conservative approach in the amount of healing time required before gait training. The protocol of this operation requires that the greater trochanter be reflected before the prosthetic implant is installed and be reinserted with an internal fixation device. The osteotomized bone could be damaged if stresses such as those generated by the gluteus maximus during gait were allowed to occur. A greater delay and caution in gait training is therefore warranted, and active or resisted abduction for the purpose of strengthening the gluteus medius muscle during rehabilitation should be avoided. The porous coated arthroplasties require partial weightbearing with assistive devices for a longer time to allow for bony ingrowth into the prosthetic device to occur.[8] Crutches or a walker may be necessary for as much as 6 to 9 months postoperatively, even though these candidates are generally younger and capable of more activity.

Table 6-2. THR Gait-Training Protocol

Arthroplasty	Conventional (Cemented THR)	Bipolar Osteonics Ingrowth	Porous Coated	Trochanteric Osteotomy[a]
Mobilize (out of bed)	Postoperative day (POD) 1–2	POD 2	POD 2	POD 2–5
Ambulation weightbearing	Partial weightbearing (PWB) to weightbearing as tolerated at discharge	(Porous coated stem, bipolar head) PWB 40–50 lbs.	PWB 40–50 lbs.	PWB
Range of motion of hip flexion	Same criteria for all: POD 2 up to 30°, POD 4–6 up to 60°, POD 6–10 up to 90°.			
Precautions	Applies to all: Avoid dislocation forces at hip, which is a combination of hip flexion, adduction, and internal rotation. No hip flexion greater than 90°.		No resisted abduction of hip. Initially walk with a slightly abducted gait.	

[a] No active abduction.
(From K. Lawrence, orthopaedic team supervisor of Physical Therapy Department, Medical College of Virginia, Richmond, VA, with permission.)

Gait training typically begins in the parallel bars. The patient assumes the standing posture either through the use of a tilt table or through instructions in sit-to-stand technique from the wheelchair. Many postoperative patients, particularly the elderly owing to their impaired circulation, experience temporary postural hypotension while coming to standing. This may be prevented or minimized with the use of antiembolus stockings and asking the patient to perform ankle "pumps" (see Appendix 6-2) before standing. Patients assuming a stance posture on the tilt table may be asked to flex their hips, knees, and ankles during the procedure, much like walking in place. Close guarding of the patient is necessary during gait-training activities for these patients in the early days postoperatively. Being aware that the patient's deficiencies in balance during stance or ambulation may have had a role in bringing them to their present circumstances is an important fact to keep in mind. Gait training quickly progresses to the use of a walker or, for younger patients with better balance, crutches. Instruction in stair climbing, stand-pivot transfers using chairs of different heights, the use of a raised commode seat, and getting in and out of an automobile correctly are all performance goals that should be accomplished before discharge. Patients who are unable to achieve all these activities independently during their short stay in the hospital may need to receive further inpatient therapy at rehabilitation centers or nursing homes before returning to their own homes. Pain continues to govern and modify the gait appliance used, as does the patient's balance, energy expenditure, and level of awareness.

Patients requiring bilateral total hip arthroplasties are generally scheduled for two separate surgical dates 6 months to 2 years apart. This allows the operated hip the time necessary for rehabilitation and recovery so that it may assume full weightbearing after the subsequent operation. On rare occasions, the patient receives bilateral total hip replacements in one operation. This surgical procedure places a significantly greater stress on the patient during the recovery phase. These patients are not generally let out of bed until day 2 to 5 postoperatively. The exercise and active range of motion exercise criteria remain the same. The gait pattern employed is a four-point gait with a walker or crutches, so that no more than one-half of the body weight is being borne on one leg at any given time. The concern of prosthetic subluxation for these patients prevents their sitting until after postoperative day 3.

To date there has been little reported research on physical therapy's role in the rehabilitation management of THR patients and their ambulatory status. Barnes[16] studied the factors associated with the ability to achieve prefracture ambulatory status in 70 inpatients in a geriatric rehabilitation center. The researcher noted in retrospect that factors such as the patient's orientation, alertness, and motivation were difficult to operationalize in this study. As is true in causal comparative studies, other extraneous variables not mentioned in the study could have had a significant impact on the outcome of ambulation status for these patients. The researcher did conclude, based on his findings, that clinicians can expect 40 to 50 percent of fracture patients over the age of 70 to achieve prefracture ambulatory status after 60 or more physical therapy visits. Not all the patients mentioned in this study received the THR procedure; many had surgery involving plates, pins, and screws for fracture stabilization. Further research specifically investigating the rehabilitation of THR patients is necessary and should be encouraged.

During the inpatient rehabilitation phase, instruction in the functional performance of activities of daily living of the THR patient is critical. The workplace and home environment of the patient will have to be adjusted to meet the demands of ambulation with an assistive device and restrictions resulting from limited range of motion of the artificial hip, limitations in energy expenditure, and safety needs. Hospitals with occupational therapy departments are fortunate in having professionals specifically trained in addressing the THR patient's adaptive equipment needs while performing home and workplace assessments. The social services departments can provide additional insight into the THR

Table 6-3. Home Care Instructions for THR Patients

Posture/Gait	Activity
First 6 Weeks Postoperatively	
1. *DO NOT* sit in low chairs.	1. *DO NOT* try to force your leg to bend at the hip in an effort (e.g., putting on your shoe and sock). Use your shoe-horn and stocking aid *between your knees.*
2. Continue to sleep on your back and do not try to sleep on your side.	
3. *DO NOT* discard crutches, walker, or cane until 12 weeks after your operation. You must be partial weightbearing during this time.	2. *DO NOT* do exercises to restore hip movement unless directed by your physical therapist. Movement will gradually return to the hip with activity and the passage of time.
4. When sitting or lying, *DO NOT* cross your legs.	
5. When reaching down to the floor, put your leg straight out behind you.	3. *DO NOT* discard the elastic stockings until at least 3 weeks after the operation, and then only if the legs aren't swelling or tiresome.
6. Lie face down on your stomach or flat on your back for 20 minutes each morning and evening.	4. *DO NOT* drive.
	5. Avoid gardening.
	6. *DO NOT* climb into a bath; sponge bathe or use a shower only.
After the First 6 Weeks	
1. You may sleep on your side.	1. *DO NOT* try to force movement of the hip by passive movements.
2. Continue partial weightbearing for additional 6 weeks unless instructed otherwise by physician.	
3. Continue daily lying face down on your stomach or flat on your back.	
In the Long Term	
1. Remember that, even if it feels normal, your hip is artificial and repetitive, over-vigorous use—such as running—is unwise. With sensible use, the joint should last for years.	
2. If you should develop an infection anywhere, contact your doctor immediately. Prompt treatment will prevent a spread of infection to the hip joint.	
3. Preventive antibiotic cover is wise if you undergo dental treatment, since it is sometimes associated with the release of bacteria into the bloodstream.	

(From D. Yarreu, physiotherapist supervisor, Princess Elizabeth Orthopaedic Hospital, Exeter, England, with permission.)

patient's home and work environments. In hospitals in which these professionals are not present or available, the responsibility for assessing the outpatient needs of the patients rests with the physical therapist. Community services, home health agencies, and private volunteer organizations are other outside resources that may be called on to answer the needs of these patients. Therapists are encouraged to develop a listing of these community organizations to be shared with patients and family members when discharge back to the community is imminent.

At the time of inpatient hospital discharge, outpatient rehabilitation is scheduled as needed. As mentioned before, many elderly patients require a longer time for rehabilitative care and supervision. Consequently, these patients may be transferred to appropriate care facilities where rehabilitation will continue until the maximal potential in functional performance is achieved. Younger, more active patients are instructed to avoid activities that would place undue forces or stresses on the THR such as contact sports, running, horseback riding, etc. These instructions will vary depending on the treatment protocol used. Table 6-3 is an example of an instruction sheet developed for THR patients that is reviewed and given to them at the time of discharge. This particular protocol emphasizes the activities, postures, and gait patterns that should be followed and those that should be avoided. The instructions also delineate the differences of rehabilitation activities during the first 6 weeks, after 6 weeks, and over the long term.

Complications Affecting Rehabilitation

As previously noted, patient complications seen during the first few days after surgery include thrombophlebitis, pressure sores, pneumonia, and postanesthetic confusion. With proper awareness and prompt attention by the medical and rehabilitation teams, these complications can be minimized and avoided. The more troubling complications in THR procedures occur in the weeks, months, and years following the surgery and involve disabling pain and prosthetic failure.

Two recently reported studies analyzed the clinical results of THR patients from two perspectives. In the first study, the authors investigated patients who underwent THR using the porous coated femoral implants designed for biologic fixation.[9] The 2-year analysis examined 307 cases; the 5-year results involved 89 cases. Successful fixation by bony ingrowth was reported in 93 percent of the cases in which a press fit type of femoral stem was used. In the 2-year follow-up, occasional pain and antalgic gait were reported by 14 and 21 percent of the subjects, respectively. A 10-year follow-up from 1969 through 1980 on 791 hip arthroplasties done with the Charnley, Muller, or Trapezoidal-28 (T-28) prostheses was investigated by Merrell and associates.[17] Women and older patients were found to have the best implant survival rates. Reported implant success after 10 years was 91 percent for the Charnley prosthesis, 88 percent for T-28, and 80 percent for the Muller prosthesis. The investigators concluded that the smaller femoral head design of the Charnley prosthesis, accompanied by a thicker acetabular cup, allowed for greater absorption of the frictional and stress forces involved in motion.

The literature underscores two important issues to be considered in THR rehabilitation. First, it appears that the two common methods of total joint implant fixation will continue to be used by orthopaedic surgeons for the near future. Second, both methods, while demonstrating improved success rates, still report a significant percentage of patients whose long-term outlook is one of pain, discomfort on ambulation, and even prosthetic failure.

Engh and Bobyn[8] describe three different forms of thigh pain symptomatology related to femoral implants. Either of the above surgical approaches may elicit these pain symptoms, but for different reasons. A successful cemented THR provides the patient, within a short interval after surgery, pain-free movement while performing routine daily activities. The artificial implant feels like an integral part of the femur. Strength and stability of the THR are perceived by the patient to be equal to the noninvolved side. If femoral component loosening occurs over time, that security and stability is lost and patients experience what is referred to as start-up pain. This type of thigh pain occurs upon immediate loading of the hip, subsides as the patient stabilizes the leg, but ultimately increases with continued activity. In a cement-fixed prosthesis, the start-up pain signifies a loosening of the PMMA bond with the femur, a precursor to prosthetic failure. In a biologic fixation, however, the investigators contend that start-up pain is a manifestation of the delayed bony ingrowth necessary for stability and strength.[9] Therapists are instructed to keep these patients on crutches longer than the normally expected time. In some patients who have received a porous coated implant and are experiencing start-up pain, this symptom will totally disappear over several months of partial weightbearing.

Another type of thigh pain, different in character, is referred to as end pain because it occurs in the thigh at a location corresponding to the end of the femoral stem of the prosthesis. End pain is milder than start-up pain and is experienced only after several hours of activity. Radiographs usually show signs of good fixation of the proximal isthmus of the femoral component but motion between the stem and the femur distally. Cyclic compression of the femoral cortex against the stem, as seen in walking, is thought to evoke end pain. This pain is only reported in the literature referring to biologic fixation procedures. End pain is more difficult to correct and may result in the patient's long-term use of a cane or crutches when loading the prosthesis for several hours.

Fatigue fracture pain usually occurs during the bone-remodeling stage of 3 to 6 months and is seen in elderly patients with large intramedullary canals, thin cortices, and large-diameter femoral stems. Fatigue fracture pain occurs in the mid-thigh region and is experienced upon initial loading. Unlike start-up pain, this symptom does not decrease with a few steps and will require the use of crutches or a cane for partial weightbearing. Radiographic appearance shows no periosteal reaction and is that of a well-fixed prosthesis. In porous coated implants, a period of restricted activity generally will result in the subsiding of fatigue fracture pain.

The ultimate failure of the femoral component of a THR may occur as a result of falls, dislocations, or defects in the implant. Cup arthroplasties are known to wear out over time also, owing to frictional stresses placed on portions of the acetabular cup during repetitive loading conditions. Revision or replacement surgery may be attempted. Revision procedures of the cup have recently met modest success, but the femoral component replacement is still not a viable alternative owing to the loss of bone stock.[5] Faced with the poor prognosis for implant replacement, the reader can understand the recent interest in biologic implants that promise greater long-term success, especially for the younger THR candidate.

Rehabilitation after Open Reduction Internal Fixation of Hip Fractures

Not all hip fractures in the elderly patient necessitate a total joint replacement. Indeed, THR for elderly fracture patients is only indicated when joint function is also compromised or called into question. Likewise, some patients are not able to withstand the extensive physical demands of a THR, so less traumatic surgical intervention is indicated.

Fractures, referred to anatomically at the hip, in fact may arise at sites from the acetabulum, head of the femur, and intertrochanteric, trochanteric, and subtrochanteric lines. They are surgically treated with the use of various pins, plates, rods, nails, and screws designed to provide relative immobility while resisting the forces of tension, bending, and torsion. It is not within the scope of this chapter to review each surgical device or procedure currently in use today. Nevertheless, some aspects of the types of hip fracture and surgical repair have direct bearing on physical therapy and rehabilitation and are briefly discussed.

Hip fracture management for all populations, but especially the elderly, has changed significantly in the past 40 years. Previous conservative treatment involving closed reduction, hip spica casting, and lengthy bed immobilization has given way to direct surgical intervention. Although open reduction internal fixation (ORIF) carries a number of dangers, such as infection or anesthetic reaction, nevertheless, research has shown that mortality and morbidity statistics are substantially diminished with ORIF as opposed to the more conservative measures.[18] Postfracture psychosis seen in the elderly is reported to be greater in those patients consigned to long bed rest regimens.[19] For elderly patients who have sustained hip fractures, it is commonly understood among orthopaedic surgeons that, barring any complications, the ideal time for ORIF is within 24 to 48 hours of the fracture.[19]

Hip fractures are divided into two major types: those involving the trochanteric region and those found in the intracapsular portion of the femoral neck. The wide, cancellous bone stock found at the trochanteric level provides fractures of this type an excellent prognosis because of the reparative potential and adequate blood supply. Fractures of the intracapsular portion of the femoral neck on the other hand show a greater instance of delayed union or nonunion because of the poor vascular supply to the head of the femur and the limited amount of cancellous bone. Anderson[19] reports that fully 30 percent of fractures of this type ultimately result in avascular necrosis owing to the compromised blood supply to the femoral head.

As a rule, physical therapy does not play a role in preoperative assessment or instruction of hip fracture patients scheduled to receive an ORIF procedure. Immediate postoperative rehabilitation at bedside concentrates on providing and instructing the patient in bed mobility while maintaining proper alignment of the operative limb.[15] Patients are instructed to lie flat on their back for 1 hour every day to avoid developing hip flexor contractures. Forced hip flexion or rotation is to be avoided at all costs; therefore, patients are discouraged from twisting forward or to either side in their beds for the first 7 to 10 days postoperatively. Patients are allowed to assume a semireclined position after 24 hours and are assisted into protectively positioned side lying as soon as possible. Generally this occurs with the nurse's or therapist's assistance 2 to 3 days postoperatively. The side-lying position greatly aids in the patient's toiletry and pulmonary postural drainage and the prevention of decubitus ulcers. An overhead trapeze is essential for fractured hip patients during the first few days postoperatively, since all their bathing and toiletry occurs at bedside. Frankel and Nordin[20] report that forces of up to four times body weight were found to act on the hip when the patient used elbows and heels to elevate the hips while being placed on a bedpan. These forces are greatly reduced with the use of an overhead trapeze.

Patients receiving ORIF generally are not placed on active or passive exercise regimens since the purpose of the surgery is to promote bone healing through the artificial stabilization of the fracture fragments by internal fixation. Unlike the casted Co-Cr-Mo alloy used in THR, 316L stainless steel is the preferred material for most internal fixation devices. Although more corrosive over time, 316L steel does provide greater resistance to higher stresses without breaking. While demonstrating a high modulus of elasticity, the corrosive nature of this alloy explains why these devices may need to be removed over time. After instruction in proper transfer techniques, these patients are generally brought to the department for instruction in gait training and adapted activities of daily living. A number of researchers point out that a non-weightbearing gait pattern places a greater load on the hip joint than a touch-down gait because the muscles around the hip must contract to carry the weight of the limb in non-weightbearing.[20–22] A non-weightbearing gait pattern is demonstrated by these researchers to take about 80 percent of the load off the hip joint, compared with 90 or 95 percent load reduction with a toe touch gait. Like the THR patient, elderly hip fracture patients receiving an ORIF will generally use a walker, or crutches if their balance and mobility are exceptional. Over 12 to 16 weeks the gait pattern will evolve into partial weightbearing to weightbearing as tolerated, based on the surgical procedure, area of the fracture, radiographic findings of anatomic healing, and patient comfort. The patient eventually advances to the use of a straight cane, which is reported to relieve approximately 60 percent of the load on the hip during the stance phase of gait.[20]

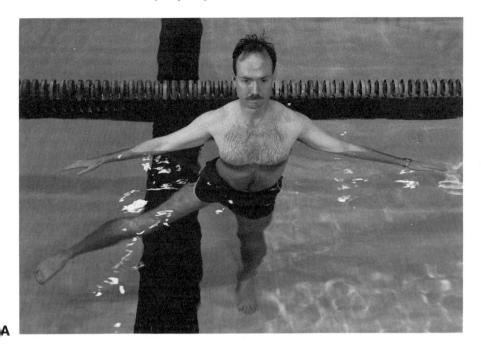

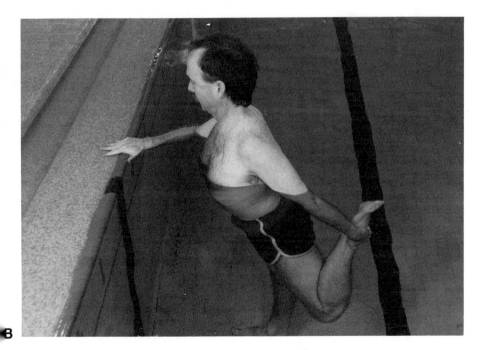

Fig. 6-1. **(A & B)** Pool exercises for the postoperative fracture patient.

As healing occurs over time, patients are encouraged to perform active exercises through a comfortable range. Since most patients have been discharged from physical therapy services by this time, they are often at a loss in finding resources to assist them in regaining function, strength, and balance. Many organizations such as the YMCA or local clubs have developed aerobic classes designed for the elderly. With proper supervision and guidance, these organizations provide an excellent avenue for the long-term rehabilitation of the elderly patient with a fractured hip. Figure 6-1 gives examples of pool exercises that allow the postoperative fracture patient to regain strength, proprioceptive sense, and mobility in a reduced gravity environment.

Johnston and Schmidt[23] did a detailed study assessing the mean measures of maximum hip motion required during common activities. They found that simple activities such as tying a shoe with the foot on the floor required 124° of hip flexion; ascending a stair required 67° of flexion; while sitting down on a chair required 104° of flexion on average. While certain activities are adapted, as they were for THR patients, over the long term patients will find a need for this amount of excursion as their mobility increases.

One school of thought believes that, regardless of the site of the hip fracture, elderly patients should receive a THR procedure because of the speed of recovery in function and lessened medical complications. This notion has been disputed by other researchers who show that patients receiving ORIF for fracture management have similar lengths of hospital stay.[24] One incontrovertible fact, however, was that THR patients were generally ambulating with greater mobility and weightbearing sooner than patients receiving conventional surgery. Recent advances in the development of the Pugh nail procedure may have changed this disparity. Over a 3-year period, Malkin and associates[24] found that the 445 patients who received the Pugh nail process had extremely low complication rates, rapid achievement of functional status, and reduced hospital stay. This operative procedure allows patients to ambulate (toe touch gait pattern) as early as the third day, with weightbearing as tolerated allowed soon after. The researchers thought that this early return to ambulation maintained the patient's skill in walking and independence.

SUMMARY

The successful rehabilitation program for hip fracture candidates should consider the following points:

1. A concerted, cooperative effort at communication and sharing of complementary goals and objectives between all members of the medical rehabilitation team is essential for successful outcomes.

2. The preoperative examination and instruction sessions greatly enhance the physical therapist's ability to plan a realistic rehabilitation program for the THR patient. The patients demonstrate better awareness, compliance, and motivation during the rehabilitation sessions postoperatively if they understand

what is expected of them, when goals have been set with their input, and when their abilities are taken into consideration.

3. Final performance outcomes should be considered in a functional context for each individual patient, with a pain-free postsurgical hip and no weakness or hesitation in function the ultimate measures of success.

Further clinical research into the factors and variables that will predict rehabilitation success in hip fracture patients is sorely needed. A better understanding of variables such as age, physical performance status, motivation, orientation, and disease state would provide the physical therapist and other practitioners a clearer picture in projecting final outcomes. This would enhance the role of physical therapy in the rehabilitation of all fractured hip patients and lead to improved outcomes for those patients.

ACKNOWLEDGMENTS

I acknowledge the graphics by Deborah Miller and photography by Alex Leidholdt at Old Dominion University.

REFERENCES

1. Jennings JJ, Gerard F: Total hip replacement in patients with rheumatoid arthritis. South Med J 71:1112, 1978
2. Opitz JL: Total joint arthroplasty: Principles and guidelines for postoperative physiatric management. Mayo Clin Proc 54:602, 1979
3. Wong J, Wong S: A randomized controlled trial of a new approach to preoperative teaching and patient compliance. Int J Nurs Stud 22:105, 1985
4. Walker PS, Eng C: Human Joints and Their Artificial Replacements. p. 254. Charles C Thomas, Springfield, IL, 1977
5. Turek S: Orthopaedics: Principles and Their Applications. 4th Ed. p. 1141. JB Lippincott, Philadelphia, 1984
6. Cochran GV: A Primer of Orthopedic Biomechanics. p. 122. Churchill Livingstone, New York, 1982
7. Kumar V, Redford JB: Rehabilitation of hip fractures in the elderly. Am Fam Physician 29:173, 1984
8. Engh CA, Bobyn JD: Biological Fixation in Total Hip Arthroplasty. p. 228. Slack, Thorofare, NJ, 1985
9. Engh CA, Bobyn JD, Glassman AH: Porous-coated hip replacement: The factors governing bone ingrowth, stress shielding, and clinical results. J Bone Joint Surg 69:145, 1987
10. Coventry MB: The 1988 Yearbook of Orthopedics. p. 114. Year Book Medical Publishers, Chicago, 1988
11. Alkire MJ, Dabezies EJ, Hastings PR: High vacuum as a method of reducing porosity in polymethylmethacrylate. Orthopedics 10:1533, 1987
12. Lidgren L, Bodelind B, Moller J: Bone cement improved by vacuum mixing and chilling. Acta Orthop Scand 57:27, 1987

13. Brady LP: A multifaceted approach to prevention of thromboembolism: A report of 529 cases. South Med J 70:546, 1977
14. Ley P, Bradshaw PW, Eaves D, Walker CM: A method for increasing patients' recall of information presented by doctors. Psych Med 3:217, 1973
15. Powell M: Orthopaedic Nursing and Rehabilitation. 9th Ed. p. 583. Churchill Livingstone, Edinburgh, 1986
16. Barnes B: Ambulation outcomes after hip fracture. Phys Ther 80:317, 1984
17. Merrell A, Campbell R, Campbell ED: Long-term comparison of the Charnley, Muller and Trapezoidal-28 total hip prosthesis: A survey analysis. J Arthroplasty 2:299, 1987
18. Crenchaw AH: Campbell's Operative Orthopaedics. Vol. 1. p. 9. CV Mosby, Saint Louis, 1971
19. Anderson RL: Conservative treatment of fractures of the femur. J Bone Joint Surg 49-AL:1371, 1967
20. Frankel VH, Nordin M: Basic Biomechanics of the Skeletal System. p. 168. Lea & Febiger, Philadelphia, 1980
21. Radin EL, Simon SR, Rose RM, Paul IL: Practical Biomechanics for the Orthopedic Surgeon. p. 119. Wiley Medical Publishers, New York, 1979
22. Evans FG: Biomechanical Studies of the Musculoskeletal System. p. 64. Charles C Thomas, Springfield, IL 1961
23. Johnston RC, Schmidt GL: Hip motion measurements for selected activities of daily living. Clin Orthop 72:205, 1970
24. Malkin S, Frankenburg F: Fractures of the hip: A three year survey in one hospital, including experience with the Pugh nail procedure. J Am Geriatr Soc 26:506, 1978

APPENDIX 6-1

Total Hip
Replacement Exercises

Patient Name_____   Therapist _____

  Physician_____

Do Only Exercises Checked

Exercise   **Repetitions**

1. In slings or springs, gently bounce leg.   ————

2. In slings or springs, press knee against bed. Hold for 10   ————
   seconds.

3. Gently bend hip and knee in slings.   ————

(*Continued*)

4. Swing operated leg outward in slings. Do *not* cross the midline when bringing leg inward.

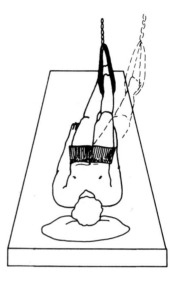

————

5. With roll under knee, lift heel off bed while knee remains on roll. *CAUTION:* Knee must stay on the roll. Hold for 10 seconds.

————

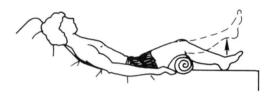

6. With towel around thigh, assist hip and knee bending by pulling towel gently to the point of tenderness.

————

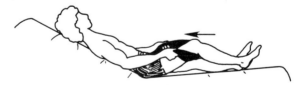

7. Lie flat on back. Slide operated leg outward on the bed. Do *not* cross midline when bringing leg inward.

————

(From B. Salmon, staff physiotherapist: Orthopaedic and Arthritic Hospital, Toronto, Canada, with permission.)

APPENDIX 6-2

Total Hip
Exercise Program

General Instructions:

Unless otherwise indicated, the following exercises are to be done lying flat on your back on a firm surface. Do only those exercises checked for you. Do them slowly.

Ankle pumps: Pump feet up and down as far as possible. Repeat _____ times, _____ times a day.

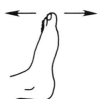

Quad sets: With leg straight, toes pointing up, tighten your thigh muscles and straighten your knee. Hold 5 seconds then relax. Repeat _____ times, _____ times a day.

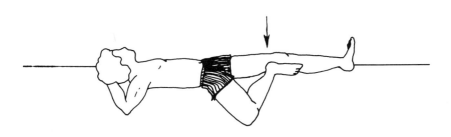

Gluteal sets: Squeeze the buttocks together, hold 5 seconds, then relax. Repeat _____ times, _____ times a day.

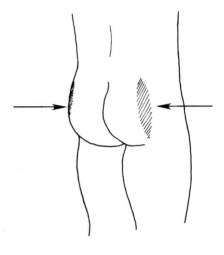

Hamstring sets: Bend operated leg slightly. Pull heel into bed without moving leg. Hold 5 seconds, then relax. Repeat _____ times, _____ times a day.

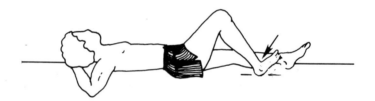

Alternate hip hiking or *"hula" exercise:* With legs straight and toes up: push one leg down towards the foot of the bed while pulling the other leg up. Alternate legs. Repeat _____ times, _____ times a day.

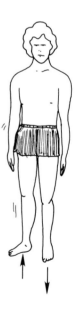

Half bridge: Bend nonoperated leg, foot resting flat on bed. Keep operated leg straight. Slowly raise buttocks as high as possible, hold 5 seconds, then slowly lower buttocks. Repeat _____ times, _____ times a day.

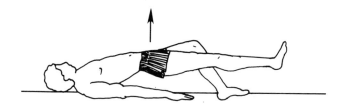

Hip flexor stretch: Pull nonoperated knee to chest and push operative leg long and into bed. Hold 15 seconds, then relax. Repeat _____ times, _____ times a day.

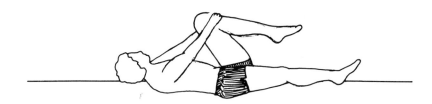

Hip flexion: Slowly bend the operated leg, sliding the heel up toward the buttocks. *DO NOT* bend hip further than 90 degrees. Repeat _____ times, _____ times a day.

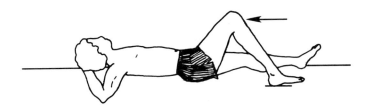

Active abduction: With legs straight and toes up, slide operated leg out to side. *DO NOT* cross leg over midline when returning leg to the starting position. Repeat _____ times, _____ times a day.

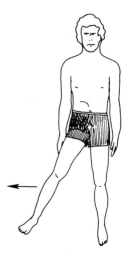

(From K. Lawrence, orthopaedic team supervisor, Physical Therapy Department, Medical College of Virginia, Richmond, VA, with permission.)

7 | Physical Therapy Management of Nonsurgical Hip Problems in Adults

Evangeline Yoder

Major etiologic categories for classification of nonsurgical hip disorders in adults include the degenerative joint diseases, soft tissue lesions, and trauma that may result in soft tissue disorder or possibly even joint dislocation. Routine anteroposterior and lateral oblique radiographs are considered obligatory for definitive medical diagnosis of a hip disorder. To assess the integrity of the joint, both hips should be radiographed for comparison studies, and in some cases additional diagnostic tests will be required.[1] Hip disorders arising secondary to other major disease processes such as tumor, cerebrovascular accident, and vascular and paralytic conditions are not included for discussion in this chapter.

Degenerative arthrosis accounts for the largest number of nonsurgical adult hip patients treated by the physical therapist.[2,3] Demographically, primary arthritis of the hip has been found to occur with an especially high frequency in the European-American white population[4] when compared with certain Oriental and black groups, and this finding is presumably not explicable on the basis of differences in biomechanical joint loading patterns between cultures. Hoaglund et al.[4] concluded from their comparative study of hip diseases that primary arthritis may be a "disease of the European-American white population" whose cause is unknown. Although total hip replacement for moderate and advanced stages of arthrosis is now well established, there exist a significant number of patients who fall short of meeting surgical criteria but suffer sufficient dysfunction to require conservative treatment.

Soft tissue lesions of the hip may be categorized according to the type of tissues they involve—contractile tissues, noncontractile tissues, or both.[5,6] Contractile tissues are the muscle belly, its tendon, the musculotendinous junction, and the tendinous-periosteal junction. Insert (noncontractile) soft tissue lesions of the hip may involve the joint capsule, ligaments, fascia, bursae, or nerves.

Discussions in this chapter focus on basic considerations for treatment planning and review the following patient management strategies: passive joint mobilization; thermal and electrical modalities; soft tissue syndrome treatment protocols; exercise methods; pool therapy; and gait and functional training for the adult with nonsurgical hip disorder.

CONSIDERATIONS FOR TREATMENT PLANNING

Clinical evaluation of the patient with hip disorder requires that the spine, pelvis, and distal limb segments also be examined. Fundamental goals of the clinical evaluation are to reproduce the patient's signs and symptoms and to localize their true site of origin.[5-7] Since the lumbar spine frequently refers symptoms to the hip and buttock areas, examination must rule out the contribution of distal sites to the clinical picture.[6] Treatment can be optimally effective only if it is preceded by accurate analysis of the underlying cause of the dysfunction.

Patient Problem List

Chapter 2 of this text and many other sources[1,5-11] discuss the content areas and specific tests that should be included in the clinical evaluation of the patient with a hip disorder. The completed evaluation will provide the data base for generation of a problem list. The subjective (S) and objective (O) portions of the evaluation should provide answers to the following questions:

1. Where is the site of origin for signs and symptoms? (Are symptoms localized? Referred? Both? Symptoms cannot be reproduced?)
2. Which types of tissue are implicated (contractile, noncontractile, or both)?
3. What is the most probable cause of the patient's current dysfunction (specific precipitating incidents or circumstances; recent life crises; life-style patterns; other)?
4. What is the overall impact of dysfunction on the patient's functional abilities and life-style (cosmetic; nuisance; total incapacitation)?

The dysfunction analysis or problem list forms the basis for establishing goals of treatment that are measurable and functional.[12,13] When using the SOAP format (subjective, objective, assessment, plan) for written documentation, the problem list fits logically and sequentially into the assessment (A) section.

The Treatment Plan

One or more treatment goals should be formulated for each area of dysfunction identified on the patient problem list. Each goal should then be further defined by a stated subset of measurable behavioral objectives. A behavioral objective must include the following information[14,15]:

1. *Who* is to accomplish the behavior? The patient . . .
2. *What* is to be accomplished? . . . will walk with Lofstrand crutches . . .
3. Under what *conditions?* . . . pain-free on level ground using a two-point gait . . .
4. Using what quantitative and/or qualitative *measurement criteria?* . . . for a distance of 40 yards in 10 minutes.

Measurable treatment objectives must be defined to describe patient status, document changes in performance, and predict realistic goals.[16] The treatment plan is the result of the evaluation process. The selection of appropriate treatment strategies is subsequently based on the identified individual needs and goals agreed on with the patient.

PASSIVE JOINT MOBILIZATION PROCEDURES

Passive joint mobilization procedures are most often indicated for the nonsurgical hip patient who suffers pain and movement limitation from degenerative arthritis. Severe pain and limitation of movement may occur early in the disease despite the absence of significant bony changes on radiographs. Conservative treatment can frequently diminish symptoms and restore function in these patients.[2,3,17]

The documented causes of osteoarthritis are numerous. In addition to aging, hip pathologies such as coxa valga, avascular necrosis, or incongruity or instability of the joint may be precipitating causes.[1,17,18] Fibrotic thickening of the joint synovial tissue and overlying fibrous capsule with adhesion and obliteration of synovial pockets are end results of the disease process, which is initiated by a chronic reactive hyperemia of the synovium in response to the presence of degenerated cartilage in the joint cavity.[17]

The primary role of the hip joint is to provide stability for weightbearing and functional ambulation; however, normal physiologic ranges of movement are

Table 7-1. Hip Joint Characteristics

Structural classification:	Unmodified ovoid joint (ball and socket)
Degrees of freedom:	Three degrees (sagittal, frontal, transverse plane motion)
Close-packed position (maximal congruence):	Extension (E), slight abduction (AB), slight internal rotation (IR)
Loose-packed position (resting/neutral position):	Flexion (F) 30°, AB 30°, and external rotation (ER) 15°
Capsular pattern (proportional limitation):	IR > E > AB > F > ER
Ranges of movement (osteokinematic/ physiologic):	F 0–120°; E 0–15°; straight leg raise 0–100°; AB 0–45°; Adduction (ADD) 0–20°; IR 0–40°; ER 0–45°

(Data from Kaltenborn.[8])

essential for the performance of functional activities, sports, and leisure activities. Table 7-1 lists functional characteristics of the hip joint and normal ranges of movement.[8] The most stable position of the hip is the normal standing or close-packed position, that is, extension, slight abduction, and slight internal rotation.[8,19] In this position, the hip joint surfaces are maximally congruent and the anterior and inferior portions of the capsule are taut. In the patient with osteoarthritis, fibrosis and hypersensitivity are pronounced in the inferior portion of the capsule. When the patient attempts to stand, extension and abduction of the hip are likely to cause pain and spasm. The leg will tend to assume an adducted, flexed, and externally rotated position to avoid pain.[17]

In the fully established case of osteoarthritis, all movements at the hip will become restricted. The capsular pattern denotes a pattern of proportional limitation of movement for the joint[5,6,8] (Table 7-1). Internal rotation is the most limited motion, and other restrictions are listed in descending order of proportional limitation. On passive overpressure, the joint end feel is hard and unyielding.[5,6]

Types and Grades of Movement

Joint mobilizations may be performed as physiologic cardinal plane passive motions at any point in the joint range of flexion/extension, abduction/adduction, or rotation. Accessory (arthrokinematic) joint glides or joint distractions are usually initiated from the loose-packed (neutral or resting position) position of the joint (Table 7-1). Accessory movements and distractions mobilize primarily inert tissues. Physiologic movements may be used to mobilize both contractile and noncontractile tissues.

Maitland[7,20] has defined grades of joint mobilization of varying amplitudes (Fig. 7-1). Grades I to IV are termed mobilizations that are often performed as oscillatory-type movements during treatment. Grades I and II are used mainly to treat pain, while grades III and IV aim at stretching soft tissue restriction. Physiologic movement mobilizations and accessory and distraction mobilizations may be performed at any grade indicated.

Fig. 7-1. Grading scheme for passive joint mobilizations. Mobilizations (grades I to IV) may be applied from beginning joint range through the physiologic (P) limit of the joint. Manipulation (grade V) (high-velocity, short-amplitude thrust) is usually applied at the physiologic (P) limit to the anatomic (A) limit of the joint.

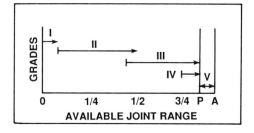

A joint manipulation may be defined as a short-duration, small-amplitude, high-velocity thrust that is applied at the physiologic (P) limit of joint range. Cyriax[5,6] has described manipulation maneuvers for shifting a "loose body" in the hip joint secondary to osteoarthritis. Sudden leg pain twinges and periodic giving way of the leg are clinical indications of the problem. Successful elimination of signs and symptoms is reportedly possible using this manipulation procedure, but recurrence of symptoms is frequent.[6]

Manipulation under anesthesia[7] is a medical procedure performed with the patient under anesthesia to restore joint range by breaking or stretching adhesions. In some orthopedic institutions, the procedure is performed on patients with mild to moderate osteoarthritic involvement of the hip and is followed by a program of active exercises (see Appendix 7-1).

When accessory joint movement glides are used to decrease hip joint capsular restriction, the direction of the appropriate glide is governed by the convex rule of mobilization. The proximal head of the femur must be glided parallel to the concave surface of the acetabulum in a direction opposite to the direction of the distal femur movement during its allied physiologic movement. For instance, if hip joint extension is restricted, the proximal head of the femur must be glided anteriorly (Fig. 7-2). If hip flexion is restricted, posterior (dorsal)

Fig. 7-2. Anterior glide (accessory movement) at the hip joint indicated for restricted hip extension.

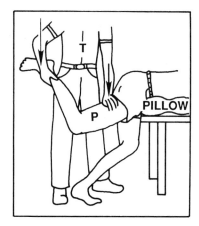

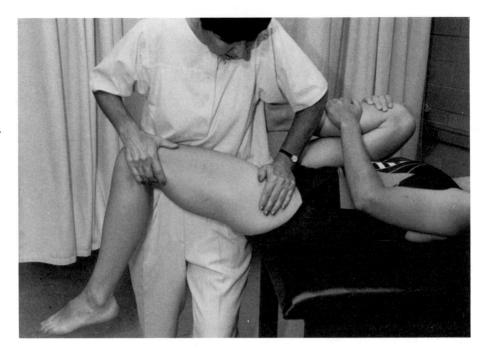

Fig. 7-3. Dorsal or posterior glide (accessory movement) at the hip joint indicated for restricted hip flexion.

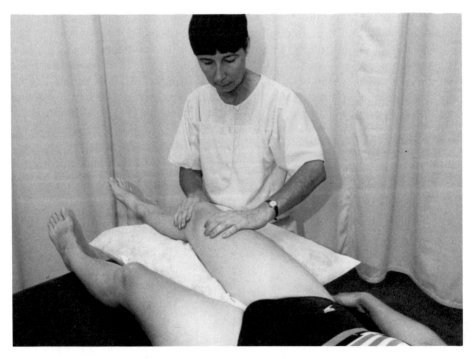

Fig. 7-4. Mobilization of the hip into internal rotation (physiologic movement) indicated for painful or restricted internal rotation.

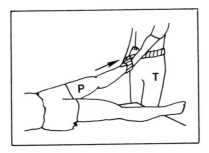

Fig. 7-5. Caudal distraction using a distal grip.

glide of the femoral head is indicated[8] (Fig. 7-3). When using physiologic joint mobilizations, however, the distal femur is moved into the direction of the restricted movement; for example, the distal femur is moved into a direction of internal rotation if internal rotation is the restricted movement[7] (Fig. 7-4).

Joint distractions are indicated for pain and any hypomobility at the hip joint and may be applied by various methods (Figs. 7-5 and 7-6). Caudal distraction is an optimal method for temporary relief of joint pain and for stretching capsular adhesion that is pronounced in the inferior portion of the joint capsule.[17]

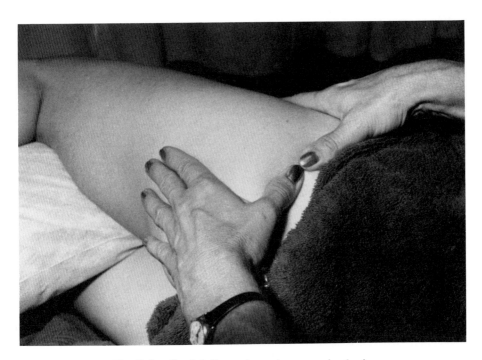

Fig. 7-6. Caudal distraction using a proximal grip.

Guidelines for Mobilization Treatment Methods

Maitland[7] has recommended guidelines for selecting mobilization treatment techniques that are based on the patient's primary dysfunction, that is, pain or joint resistance (stiffness). The acutely painful hip with severe limitation of movement should first be treated with small-amplitude accessory movements.[7,20] Guidelines for treatment progression are outlined in Table 7-2. Graded small-amplitude movements carefully applied may also be effective for reducing hip joint pain in patients with rheumatoid arthritis in subacute stages.[2]

When joint motion is less than 50 percent, but joint resistance to movement is the dominant dysfunction, physiologic movement (grade IV) to stretch the joint limitation is advocated.[7] When joint range is greater than 50 percent, treatment progresses from use of physiologic movements to use of accessory movement at the limit of the joint.

Flexion and adduction of the hip combined with simultaneous joint compression through the femur may be used to reproduce minimal signs of hip dysfunction and to assess joint end feel.[3,7,22] The flexed adducted thigh is swept through a 90° to 140° arc of flexion while maintaining joint compression. This procedure is sometimes called scouring the joint (Fig. 7-7). The normal joint end feel is a smooth arc of pain-free gliding. In an abnormal joint, pain and a bump on the arc occur during the movement. In selected nonacute cases, the procedure may be used as an effective mobilizing procedure.[3]

Theories for explaining why joint mobilizations are effective have been proposed. Grade I and II joint mobilizations may theoretically be effective in pain reduction by improving joint lubrication and circulation in tissues related to the joint.[2] Rhythmic joint oscillations also possibly activate articular and skin mechanoreceptors that play a role in pain reduction.[23,24] Grade III and IV joint distractions and stretching mobilizations may, in addition to the above-stated

Table 7-2. Guidelines for Mobilization of the Painful Hip

Examination Findings	Treatment Procedure
Pain severely limits movement (patient has less than 50% joint range)	Accessory movement (in neutral): grade I (small amplitude of movement in pain-free range)
Pain decreased	Accessory movement: grades I+ to III (increase amplitude up to grade III; increase repetitions)
Pain decreased, range increased (patient has more than 50% joint range)	Physiologic movement: grades II to III (large amplitude, short of pain)
Pain continues to decrease, range continues to increase	Physiologic movement: grades III+ to IV (push into pain)
Full range without pain	Discontinue treatment
Pain and range same (resistance limits movement)	Physiologic and accessory movements: grade IV

(Data from Van Hoesen.[21])

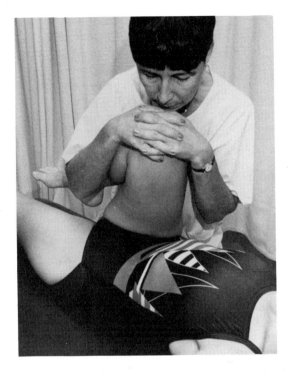

Fig. 7-7.   Combined flexion-adduction with joint compression (scouring).

effects, activate inhibitory joint and muscle spindle receptors, which aid in reducing restriction to movement.[3,23,24]

Selection of treatment procedures and treatment progression must be guided by continuous reassessment of the patient's response to a given procedure. Reassessment of patient dysfunction before, during, and after each treatment is essential.

THERMAL AND ELECTRICAL
TREATMENT MODALITIES

Thermal modalities and electrical stimulation procedures used before or after joint mobilization (and other physical therapy procedures subsequently discussed) may enhance the desired treatment effects of pain reduction and increased joint mobility. Heat modalities are widely used in treatment of degenerative joint diseases (osteoarthritis and rheumatoid arthritis) for their analgesic effects, for increasing extensibility of collagen tissue, and for decreasing muscle spasm,[25–27] but the effectiveness of some thermal modalities has been challenged.[28]

Ultrasound lends itself well for the application of heat to the hip region because of its depth of penetration and relatively few contraindications.[25,27] Ultrasound is sometimes used as a dispersion agent over a localized area after soft tissue medical injection[1] and to drive topically applied anti-inflammatory or anesthetic preparations into deeper tissues (phonophoresis).

Cryotherapy in the form of ice massage or other modes of application is reportedly effective for reduction of pain and muscle spasm.[25,28,29] Electrical stimulation may be of benefit,[25,27] and transcutaneous electrical nerve stimulation (TENS) provides at least transient relief of symptoms for acute or chronic pain in some patients.[25,30]

SOFT TISSUE SYNDROME TREATMENT PROTOCOLS

The most common soft tissue lesion syndromes about the hip that are treated by the physical therapist include bursitis, entrapment syndromes, myofascial pain and dysfunction, and muscle strains.

The three major bursae about the hip are the trochanteric, the iliopectineal, and the ischiogluteal. The usual case of bursitis results from a reactive inflammation in response to overuse or excessive pressure. Thermal modalities (heat or cold) and relief from the inciting irritation are often successful modes of conservative treatment for uncomplicated cases of bursitis.[17]

The trochanteric bursa may be irritated by an overlying tight iliotibial band. Irritation of the bursa may be caused by snapping hip, which occurs when the tensor fasciae band or tendon for the gluteal insertion slips over the trochanter during active hip flexion, adduction, or internal rotation.[1,17] Soft tissue mobilization or stretching procedures may be indicated to decrease the irritating pressure. Gluteal bursitis symptom relief may be obtained with use of ultrasound or ice locally applied and pressure relief during sitting. Possible causes of iliopectineal bursitis are osteoarthritis or iliopsoas muscle tightness. These cases may respond to stretching of the tight muscle and/or use of modalities to decrease pain.[11]

Entrapment of the lateral femoral cutaneous nerve (meralgia paresthetica) usually results from restriction imposed on the nerve by the lateral portion of the inguinal ligament. Primary symptoms are burning pain and possible numbness in the superficial anterolateral region of the thigh.[31] Heat, electrical stimulation, and evaluation for a shoe heel lift if short leg occurs on the uninvolved side are recommended as nonsurgical forms of treatment.[32]

Piriformis syndrome is the result of sciatic nerve irritation as the nerve passes under or through the muscle. Deep localized pain on active and resisted hip external rotation and pain on palpation and stretch of the hip into internal rotation are implicating signs of the disorder. Initial use of modalities followed by later use of exercise and stretch are often effective treatments.[11]

Contusion to the iliac crest secondary to athletic injury has been termed hip pointer. Bleeding, swelling, and pain result, and sometimes muscles attached to the crest may avulse. Fracture, intra-abdominal injury, or other serious injury must be ruled out. Immediate ice applications are indicated, and gentle stretching and TENS may be of benefit in later treatment of symptoms.[33]

Myofascial Pain Syndromes

Active myofascial trigger points (TPs) are foci of hyperirritability in a muscle or its fascia. Pain and/or autonomic phenomena are referred from the active TPs in patterns that are specific for the involved muscle.[34,35] Synonyms for this disorder include muscular rheumatism, myalgia, and myofascitis.[34]

The etiology of myofascial syndromes is unknown, but "nonpropagated contracture of affected muscle fibers with associated sensitization of muscle pain afferents" has been proposed to explain the characteristic presence of hard bands or nodules in involved muscles.[35] An onset of myofascial pain is often associated with acute overload stress or a chronic muscle overload. Identification of the specific TPs responsible for dysfunction through palpation, muscle stretch, and active tests is a crucial part of the patient evaluation.

Myofascial treatment techniques include stretch and spray.[34,35] Stretch and spray technique is used to inactivate TPs in the involved muscle or muscles. The patient is positioned comfortably to allow stretch of the involved muscle during simultaneous spray of the involved area with Fluori-Methane, a vapocoolant spray in the family of fluorocarbons (Freon).[34] The spray is directed at a 30° angle to the skin and applied in parallel unidirectional sweeps at a distance of 18 inches from the body surface area.[34] Precautions against spray inhalation and skin tissue damage from the vapocoolant must be observed. Patterns of pain referral for muscles around the hip have been mapped out[35] to guide the clinician when using the spray and stretch method (Fig. 7-8).

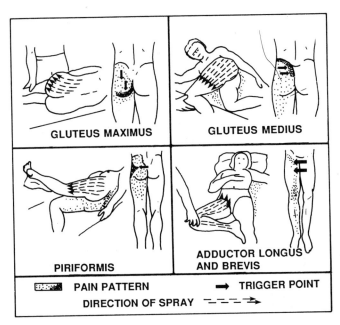

Fig. 7-8. Spray and stretch technique for selected myofascial pain syndromes in the hip region. (Modified from Simons,[35] with permission.)

The effectiveness of the stretch and spray technique for increasing hip range of motion in normal subjects has been investigated, but results are conflicting. In one study, the application of Fluori-Methane to the hamstrings of normal individuals during straight-leg-raise stretch in side-lying produced significant improvement in hip range of motion compared with control subjects who received stretch but no spray.[36] However, a second study that attempted to duplicate these results failed to demonstrate improved hip range attributable to the use of the vapocoolant spray.[37]

Soft Tissue Mobilization Procedures

Soft tissue mobilization (STM) or massage procedures are indicated for treatment of contractile and noncontractile tissue dysfunctions about the hip. In addition to traditional massage procedures (petrissage, effleurage, friction) and connective tissue massage, myofascial release procedures and STM as advocated by Barnes[38] and others[39] utilize manual manipulations to release restrictions in superficial and deep tissues. Purposes of the procedures are to decrease muscle spasm, stretch fibrous tissues, cause increased blood flow and decongestion, and improve proprioceptive awareness[39] (Figs. 7-9 and 7-10).

Effects of STM for improving hip range of motion have been reported in the

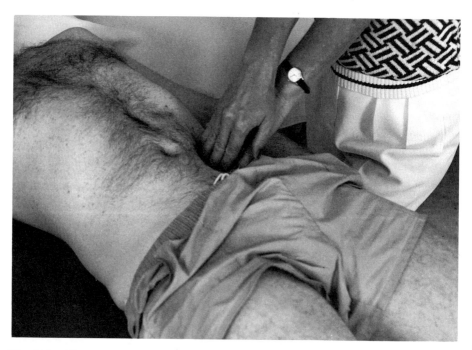

Fig. 7-9. Iliopsoas release procedure applying deep transverse pressure across the muscle belly may be indicated for a tight or painful iliopsoas muscle.

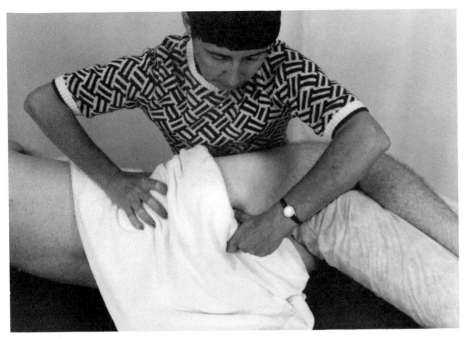

Fig. 7-10.   Piriformis soft tissue mobilization (STM) applied using firm tolerable circular movements to the painful and/or restricted muscle, or gluteals or deep rotator muscles of the hip.

literature. Crosman et al.[40] studied the effects of hamstring massage (effleurage, petrissage, friction) on hip flexion range in normal individuals and noted significant range improvements after the STM. Godges et al.[41] reported improved hip flexion and hip extension ranges in normal individuals after the application of STM to muscle groups opposing each respective motion, combined with exercise of agonistic muscles.

Muscle strain at the hip may arise insidiously or be incurred traumatically. First and second degree muscle strains are frequent injuries in sports activities. Patient history and examination reveal the nature and extent of the injury. The hamstrings are the most commonly strained muscles of the hip, especially in runners and joggers.[11,42] Strain is most likely to occur in the hamstrings during two stages of the running cycle—late forward swing and takeoff (toe off).[42,43] Strains from sports activities occur less commonly in the iliopsoas, adductor longus, and rectus femoris muscles than in the hamstrings.

Cyriax and Cyriax[6] have advocated the use of transverse friction massage for muscle or tendinous strains to maintain soft tissue mobility and prevent the formation of scars. The exact location of the injury must be identified on examination as the muscle belly or the tendon. Guidelines for positioning, treatment techniques, and precautions have been outlined in detail.[6,44] The recommended massage procedure for a hamstring strain at its proximal ischial

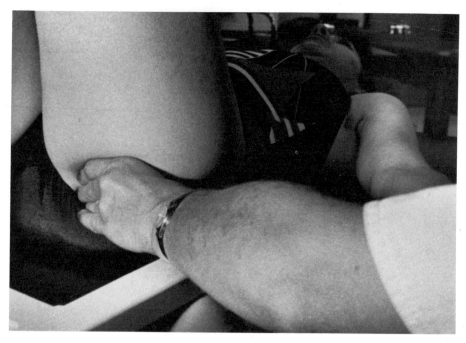

Fig. 7-11. Cyriax's transverse friction massage applied to the ischial origin of the hamstrings.

origin would place the tendon on stretch. Then strong transverse friction (nonacute case) would be applied through fixed fingers using to-and-fro movements of only the wrist and shoulder (Fig. 7-11). Acute strains may require initial rest, modality treatment, or possible medical injection.

EXERCISE PROCEDURES

Selection of exercise methods for the patient with a hip disorder is preceded by determining the status of the contractile tissues and related joint structures. Evaluation identifies the state of the muscles, the sites and causes of movement dysfunction, and the contraindications and indications for types of exercise needed. Treatment goals and objectives specify the functional context of what the muscles must do and how long they must do it. The clinician then must select appropriate methods to bring about the desired changes.[45]

Active Exercise Methods

In the patient with osteoarthritis, cardinal plane motions (see Appendix 7-1) performed isotonically are frequently used to preserve range and function of all the muscles about the hip. Positioning in extension and extension movements (Fig. 7-12) with neutral or slight internal rotation are emphasized early in treat-

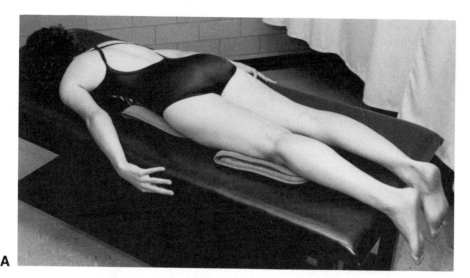

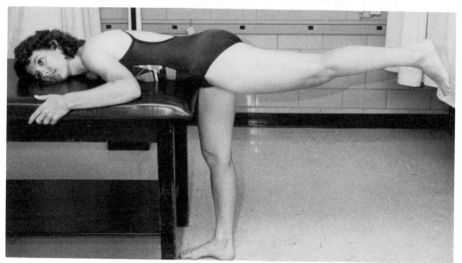

Fig. 7-12. Prevention of joint contracture. (**A**) Prone lying with hips extended in neutral rotation (20 minutes at a time). (**B**) Active hip extension with neutral rotation.

Table 7-3. Optimal PNF Patterns for Muscles of the Hip

Patterns	Muscles
Flexion-adduction-external rotation	Psoas major and minor, iliacus, pectineus, obturator externus, adductor longus and brevis, gracilis, sartorius, rectus femoris
Extension-abduction-internal rotation	Gluteus medius and minimus
Flexion-abduction-internal rotation	Tensor fasciae latae, biceps femoris
Extension-adduction-external rotation	Gluteus maximus, piriformis, obturator internus, gamellus superior and inferior, adductor magnus, semitendinosus, semimembranosus

(Data from Voss et al.[46])

ment to deter development of the typical deformity patterns of hip flexion with adduction and external rotation. The spiral diagonal patterns of proprioceptive neuromuscular facilitation (PNF) may also be used as active isotonic exercise movements. Optimal patterns of PNF to promote active contraction in muscles of the hip are summarized in Table 7-3.[46]

Active isometric exercise methods, known as isometric muscle setting, may be used for muscles at the hip when movement is contraindicated by acute pain or joint instability. Isometric contractions of hip muscles may also be performed through irradiation caused by isotonic or isometrically resisted contraction in another part of the body (Fig. 7-13). This method allows for improving or maintaining the contractile mechanism without joint movement.[46]

Active exercises are ideally performed within a functional context. Simultaneous contraction of hip extensors and abductors in weightbearing is the normal coactivation pattern used in early stance-phase gait.[47–49] Exercises and balance training in standing can be used to reinforce this pattern (Fig. 7-14). Active hip flexion with adduction, knee flexion, and dorsiflexion in standing simulates the normal swing phase of gait and promotes balance control in weightbearing on the contralateral stance leg (Fig. 7-15). Other functional exercises such as sit-stand-sit require simultaneous activation of hip muscles coordinated with other trunk and limb patterns normally used to accomplish the activity (Fig. 7-16). Advanced active exercise programs for the athlete should also incorporate activities that simulate the actual circumstances and patterns of contraction

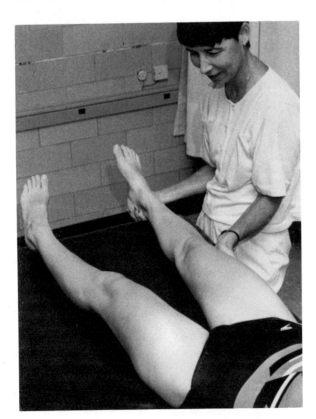

Fig. 7-13. Isometrically resisted abduction on the right elicits reflex contraction of the contralateral abductors through irradiation.

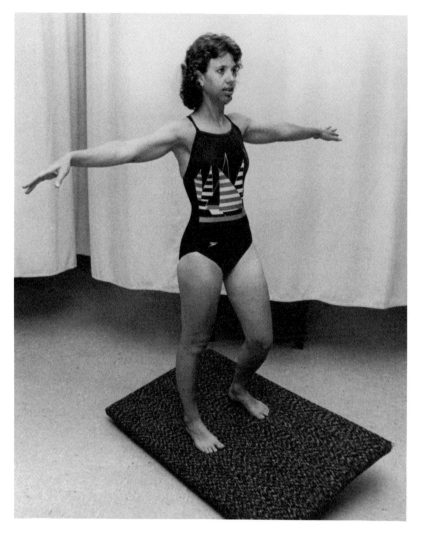

Fig. 7-14.   Use of the tilt board to promote balance and weight shift in standing. The pattern of hip extension with lateral shift of the pelvis over the right leg is demonstrated.

used in the sport.[43] Likewise, task-oriented exercise programs (work hardening) should be instituted for the patient who intends to resume a type of employment that requires a predetermined level of work performance.

A large number of patients with osteoarthritis seen for exercise programs will be over 65. The Feldenkrais[50] approach uses a program of active exercises to develop awareness through movement that provides an interesting active pain-free method for maintaining and improving functional movement of the limbs and trunk. The appropriate movement lessons should be chosen and monitored by the patient's physical therapist to ensure that the program is effective and safe. Some patients will require assessment of vital signs, especially if they have any concomitant history of blood pressure or heart problems.

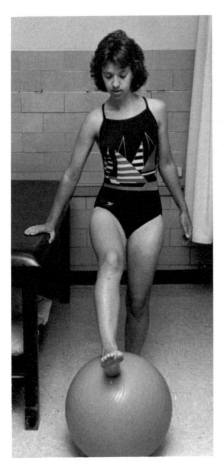

Fig. 7-15. Right leg swing-phase gait is practiced by rolling the ball forward and backward with the foot while the contralateral leg maintains unilateral stance.

Resistance Exercise Methods

Primary goals of resistance exercises are to increase strength (muscle tension), muscular endurance (low-intensity repetitive muscle performance for prolonged periods), and power (work per unit of time).[33]

Isokinetic exercise is isotonic movement performed at a fixed speed with accommodating resistance throughout the range of motion. Isokinetic equipment can be used to develop strength, power, and speed of muscle contraction. Protocols have been devised for isokinetic exercise of the hip flexors, extensors, abductors, and adductors in the standing and lying positions.

Traditional regimens of resistance exercises such as the DeLorme and Oxford methods, using externally applied weights for movements with the distal lever free, may be used to develop strength and endurance of the hip muscula-

Fig. 7-16. Sit-stand-sit practice requires concentric and eccentric control of the hip extensors in a weightbearing position used for standing up and sitting down.

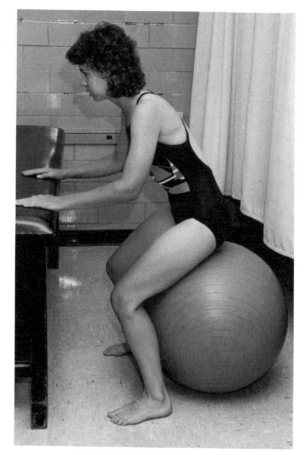

ture. The progressive resistance exercise programs utilize various types of equipment to provide external resistance.[51]

PNF patterns performed as maximally resisted isotonic motions can be considered manual isokinetic exercise—the clinician uses varying degrees of resistance throughout the range of movement to match the patient's maximal effort (Figs. 7-17 and 7-18). Optimal patterns for application of stretch, resistance, and proprioceptive joint stimuli have been outlined for each of the hip muscles (Table 7-3). The PNF patterns can also be performed isometrically against resistance at any point in the range of joint motion.

Dynamic exercises use gravity and the body weight as the resistance force against a fixed distal lever. The femur is fixed against a stool of appropriate height for the patient, and resistance to the desired muscle group at the hip is generated by elevating the pelvis and lower trunk over the distally fixed femur. Motions of hip extension, abduction, flexion, or adduction (Fig. 7-19) can be performed and sustained as an isometric contraction in the short range of the

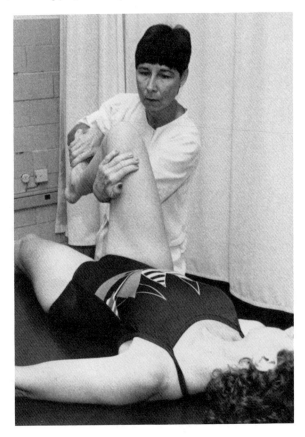

Fig. 7-17. PNF flexion-adduction pattern with isotonic manual resistance—simulates components needed for swing-phase gait.

muscle group. Bridging also utilizes body weight as a resistance force to the hip extensors and abductors. Manually applied resistance can be superimposed on the pelvis or thighs to generate maximal muscular tension in the contracting muscles (Fig. 7-20).

The stationary exercise bicycle is used to increase lower extremity strength, endurance, and range during repetitive reciprocal movements of the lower extremities (Fig. 7-21). Electromyographic analysis of lower limb muscles during pedaling has shown that the highest peak of activity for the gluteus maximus and biceps muscles as hip extensors occurred during the pedal down-stroke.[52] Stationary bicycling has also been found to be as effective for increasing range of motion at the hip joint as static stretching.[53]

The stationary bicycle is a convenient mode of exercise for home use; however, the use of vigorous protocols of cycle ergometry should be carefully

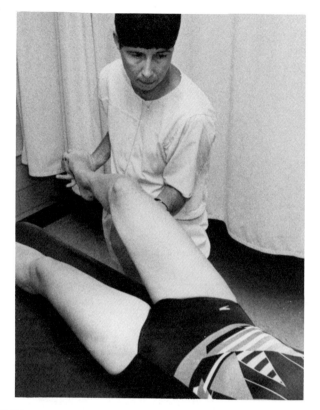

Fig. 7-18. PNF extension-abduction pattern isotonically resisted simulates hip components needed for stance-phase gait.

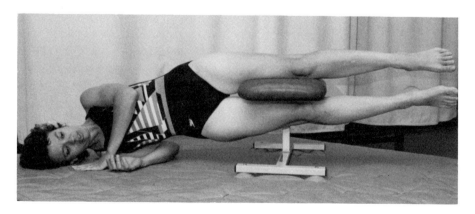

Fig. 7-19. Dynamic exercise using body weight to provide resistance for the left hip adductors.

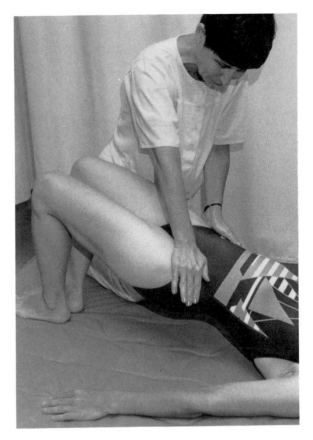

Fig. 7-20. Resisted bridging reinforces the coactivation of hip extensors with abductors and knee flexors in a weightbearing position.

monitored for cardiac effects, especially in older patients. Both blood pressure and heart rates have been found to increase markedly during this type of exercise.[54]

Stretching and Flexibility Exercises

Passive stretching (manual or mechanically applied external forces), active stretch, and self-stretching are treatment modes used to elongate the contractile tissues. Specific tests to identify tight muscles and associated tissues are standardly included on the hip evaluation. These test positions may also be used to actively or passively stretch the tight structures. For example, the Ober test position with active or externally applied force can be used to stretch tight abductors, especially the tensor fasciae latae and iliotibial band. Stretch by active or passive adduction in the standing position may also be effective (Fig.

Fig. 7-21. Stationary exercise bicycle used to promote improved hip range of motion and strength.

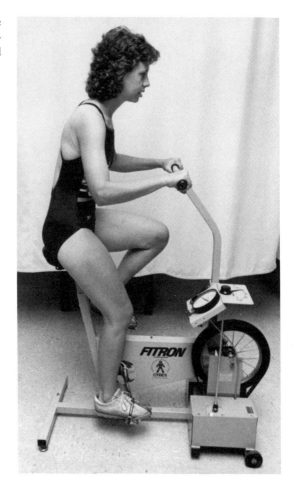

7-22).[50] Other positions that can be used to elongate tight contractile structures are the Thomas test for tight psoas or rectus femoris muscles and the straight-leg-raise (SLR) test used to assess tight hamstrings; the slump test used as a stretch technique may improve SLR range (Fig. 7-23).[56]

PNF procedures of hold-relax and contract-relax are methods of active stretching based on the Sherrington principle of successive induction.[57] The procedure demands a maximal contraction of the tight muscle into its optimal pattern (Table 7-3) after it has been placed in its maximally elongated range. According to the principle of successive induction, following a maximal contraction, the tight muscle is maximally relaxed (inhibited). Greater length following contraction of the tight muscle allows improved range of active or passive movement in the opposite direction (Fig. 7-24).

Tanigawa[58] compared the hold-relax procedure with passive mobilization of the hamstring muscles. The study demonstrated that subjects receiving the

Fig. 7-22. Iliotibial band stretch in standing.

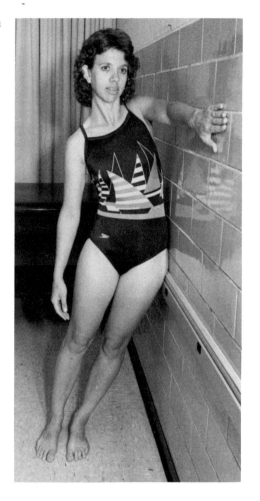

PNF procedure increased straight leg range to a higher degree and at a faster rate than did subjects receiving passive stretch. Hip flexion range during SLR was found to improve significantly in subjects receiving hold-relax and contract-relax in another study.[59] Of the two PNF techniques used (contract-relax and hold-relax), contract-relax achieved greater improvement in ranges than did hold-relax. Hold-relax utilizes only isometric contraction of all muscle components in the pattern. The contract-relax procedure uses isometric resistance to all muscles in the pattern except for the rotators; rotational components of the pattern are isotonically resisted.

Prolonged mechanical passive stretching utilizes a low-intensity external force (usually 5 to 15 pounds) applied over a long time. Weighted traction or pulley systems may be used. Loading for 20 minutes or more in an exercise session should be practiced if adequate soft tissue lengthening is to occur.[60] Limited length of the musculotendinous unit crossing a joint is responsible in

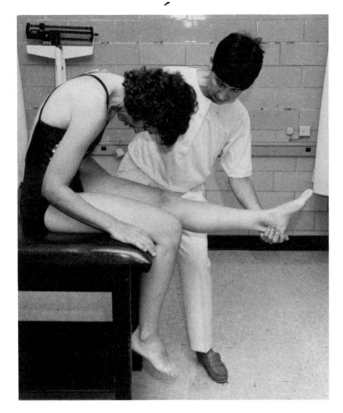

Fig. 7-23.   Hamstrings stretch using the neural tension slump test position.

many cases for diminished range. Small loads applied to tendons for long periods produce greater residual lengthening than heavy loads applied for short periods.

POOL THERAPY

The therapeutic or recreational pool provides an enjoyable and useful adjunctive medium for treatment of patients with a hip disorder. For patients with pain, movement limitation, or weightbearing limitation, the buoyant effect of water provides the advantage of diminished gravitational effects on the joints.[61,62] Modes of pool therapy for the hip patient include active exercises, stretching and resistance exercises, ambulation activities, and swimming. The mild warmth of a therapeutic pool may further contribute to the beneficial effects of movement in water.

The Medizinische Zentrum in Bad Ragaz, Switzerland, uses a pool program adapted from one developed by James McMillan in England in the 1950s, the

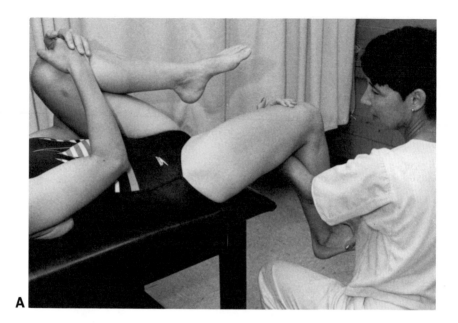

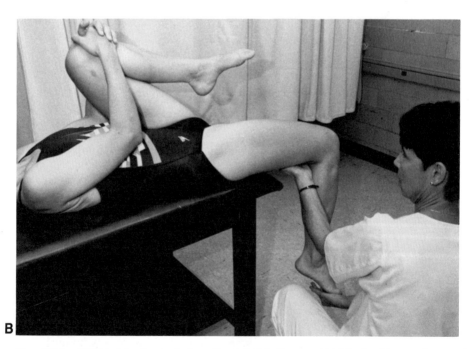

Fig. 7-24. PNF hold-relax technique for tight hip flexors. (**A**) Maximal isometric contraction into the flexion-adduction pattern is resisted. (**B**) Then, following maximal relaxation, active contraction into hip extension-abduction pattern follows (increased length of the hip flexors is achieved).

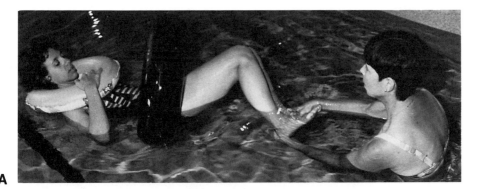

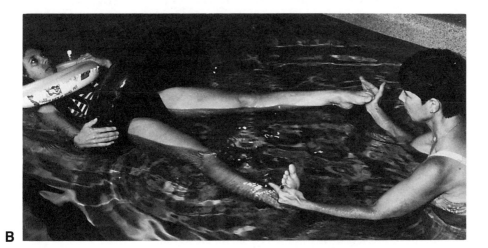

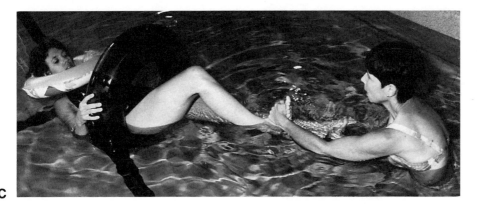

Fig. 7-25. Pool therapy: Bad Ragaz ring method. (**A**) Bilateral lower extremity flexion (isotonic resistance); (**B**) bilateral abduction with isometric resistance (flexion-abduction right leg, extension-abduction left leg); (**C**) flexion-adduction right leg (isotonic) and extension-abduction left leg (isometric).

Halliwick method.[63] Goals promoted by the program are (1) safety in water, (2) relaxation, (3) development of equilibrium and coordination, and (4) skill in a leisure activity—progression to backstroke swimming (see Appendix 7-2).

The Bad Ragaz ring method (named by the ring floats that the patient dons) is based on a modification of PNF patterns for pool use.[64] Maximal resistance, verbal commands, and joint approximation or traction are used to improve range of motion and strength in the trunk and lower limbs. Contraction patterns may be performed isotonically or isometrically (Fig. 7-25). The exercise methods are not used for patients with acute pain or for those with contraindications for resisted movement or weightbearing.

GAIT AND FUNCTIONAL ACTIVITIES TRAINING

Dysfunction factors in patients with a hip disorder that interfere with ambulation are related to biomechanical alterations during the swing and/or stance phases of gait. Problems include pain on weightbearing or movement, joint range restrictions, functional muscle weakness, leg length discrepancy, or deformity (Table 7-4). Analysis of both the stance and swing phases of gait is essential to determine the problems that must be dealt with in treatment.

Determinants of stance-phase gait involve interaction between the pelvis and hip and distal limb joints (knee and ankle) as described by Inman[47] and others.[48,49] Essential components of stance-phase gait (Fig. 7-26) include the following:

1. Lateral horizontal shift of the pelvis and trunk over the stance leg
2. Activation of the abductor mechanism on weightbearing to stabilize the hip and pelvis and prevent excessive pelvic elevation

Table 7-4. Gait Deviations Secondary to Hip Dysfunction

Gait Deviation	Possible Causes
Stance-phase gait	
Lateral trunk bend	Hip abductor weakness, hip malalignment (coxa vara, dislocation), hip pain, short leg, compensation for abducted gait
Abnormally wide base	Hip abduction contracture, joint instability, pain, leg length discrepancy
Posterior trunk bend	Hip extensor weakness
Anterior trunk bend	Quadriceps weakness combined with gluteus maximus weakness
Lordosis in stance	Hip flexion contracture, hip extensor weakness
Vaulting (normal side)	Involved side long leg and hip flexor weakness, extension ankylosis
Swing-phase gait	
Hip hiking	Long leg involved side and hip flexor weakness, contralateral short leg and hip flexion contracture
Circumduction	Hip flexor weakness, long leg swing side

(Data from New York University Medical Center.[48])

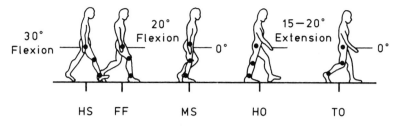

Fig. 7-26.   Stance-phase gait (sagittal plane joint components)—heel strike (HS), foot flat (FF), midstance (MS), heel off (HO), toe off (TO). (Modified from New York University Medical Center,[48] with permission.)

3. Strong activation of the hip extensors (with abductors) at heel strike into early stance—from 30° initial flexion range to approximately 20° extension at heel off

Gait-training procedures[45,65] with manual contacts at the pelvis may utilize guidance, stretch, joint approximation, and possibly resistance to promote development of appropriate patterns of control for stance-phase gait (Fig. 7-27), provided there are no contraindications (pain or instability) to weightbearing and resistance. Weight shift practice on a balance board (Fig. 7-14) and unilateral stance activities (Fig. 7-15) may also be used.

The essential components of normal swing-phase gait[47,65] (Fig. 7-28) to develop in treatment are

1. Forward rotation of the pelvis on swing-phase flexion of the hip
2. Pelvic dip (drop) of approximately 5° on the side of swing limb
3. Flexion of the hip to a maximum of 30° (activation of hip flexors) with kinematic knee flexion and dorsiflexion

Flexion patterns may be developed during contralateral limb stance activity (Figs. 7-15 and 7-27).

Pain on weightbearing is a major problem in some patients with rheumatoid hip involvement or osteoarthritis. Relief from weightbearing forces on the painful joint in standing in these patients becomes a primary aim of treatment. Quantitative and qualitative analysis of the generation of compressive forces at the hip and the muscular mechanisms involved have been thoroughly documented.[17,31,66–70] Use of a cane or crutch in the hand contralateral to the involved hip markedly decreases pressure on the hip joint. For example, pressure on the hip joint in a 150-pound person is reduced to only 120 pounds if the patient applies 30 pounds of pressure on the cane at a distance of 20 inches from the center of gravity.[31] Use of a cane on the side contralateral to the affected hip decreases the vertical and posterior components of the floor reaction force produced by the foot on the affected side.[71]

Bilateral use of canes or Lofstrand crutches may be indicated for some

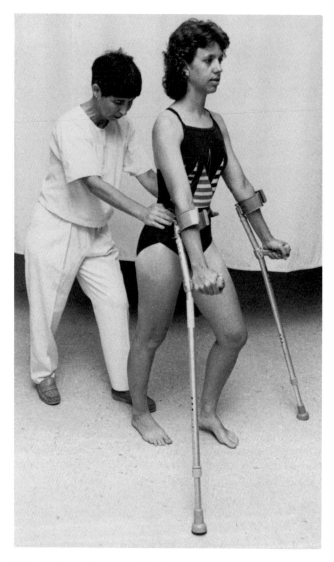

Fig. 7-27. Gait training using approximation, lateral shift of pelvis guidance on the left (stance-phase limb). Pelvic dip, forward rotation of the pelvis, and hip flexion are facilitated through manual contacts of the pelvis on the right side (swing-phase limb).

patients to further reduce weightbearing forces on the hip joint and promote a symmetric gait pattern.[62] Use of a walker for maximum functional ambulation and safety may be required for other patients.

Adoption of a special gait pattern described by Margaret Knott (course lectures in Vallejo, CA, 1971) can help to diminish pain at initial heel strike during walking. The patient is required to maximize the muscular force of the

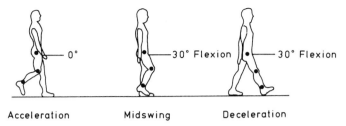

Acceleration   Midswing   Deceleration

Fig. 7-28. Swing-phase gait (sagittal plane). (Modified from New York University Medical Center,[48] with permission.)

plantar flexors during stance with avoidance of a forceful heel strike contact with the floor—called spring gait. The use of shoes with specially made cushion heels may further aid in diminishing pain on initiation of weightbearing.

The patient with leg length discrepancy should be assessed using a heel or shoe lift during walking. Shoe lifts have been reported to reduce limp, prevent undue wear on the joints, and relieve hip and back pain, but the need for use of a lift with leg length discrepancy of less than one-half inch is controversial.[72,73] Heel lifts of one-fourth inch or less are generally placed inside the shoe,[48] while higher lifts may have to be placed on the sole of the shoe.

Biomechanical requirements for joints of the lower limbs during stair climbing and descent and for other functional activities have been described in detail.[74,75] Compared with level walking, the hip joint flexes an average of 42° to 50° going up stairs, and the maximum net flexion-extension moments (in newton-meters) required for performance of stairs exceed the force requirements needed for level walking by one and one-half times. Use of a hand rail for support and negotiating stairs one step at a time (versus foot over foot) reduces the hip joint force moments significantly. These stair-climbing methods are recommended for the patient with hip pain on weightbearing.

The patient with severe and irreversible limitation of hip motion will need evaluation, training, and possible adaptive devices for the safe and functional performance of activities of daily living. Special seating devices, aids for dressing, and aids for home and leisure activities should be obtained and used as part of the treatment program.[62,76]

SUMMARY

This chapter discussed dysfunctions in the nonsurgical adult hip patient that are commonly evaluated and treated by the physical therapist. Criteria for collection of baseline clinical data and guides for establishing treatment goals and objectives were reviewed. Presentation of possible treatment strategies for patients with hip dysfunction included a description of clinical methods that may be used to meet individual patient needs.

ACKNOWLEDGMENTS

I thank Richi Ackerman, George Maihafer, and Martha Walker for assistance with the photographs, Deborah L. Miller for providing the drawings, and Stacey Hotel for typing the manuscript.

REFERENCES

1. Gordon EJ: Diagnosis and treatment of common hip disorders. Med Trial Tech Q Spring: 443, 1981
2. Grieve GP: Manual mobilizing techniques in degenerative arthrosis of the hip. Bull Orthop Section APTA 2:7, 1977
3. Grieve GP: The hip. Physiotherapy 69:196, 1983
4. Hoaglund FT, Shiba R, Newberg AH, Leung KYK: Diseases of the hip. J Bone Joint Surg 67A:1376, 1985
5. Cyriax J: Textbook of Orthopaedic Medicine. Vol. 1. Diagnosis of Soft Tissue Lesions. 8th Ed. Bailliere Tindall, London, 1982
6. Cyriax JH, Cyriax PJ: Illustrated Manual of Orthopedic Medicine. Butterworth, London, 1983
7. Maitland GD: Peripheral Manipulation. 2nd Ed. Butterworth, London, 1977
8. Kaltenborn, FM: Manual Mobilization of the Extremity Joints. 3rd Ed. Olaf Nolis Bokhandel, Oslo, 1989
9. Hoppenfeld S: Physical Examination of the Spine and Extremities. Appleton-Century-Crofts, East Norwalk, CT, 1976
10. Cookson JC, Kent BE: Orthopedic manual therapy—an overview. Part 1. The extremities. Phys Ther 59:135, 1979
11. Saudek CE: The hip. p. 347. In Gould JA, Davies GJ (eds): Orthopaedic and Sports Physical Therapy. CV Mosby, St. Louis, 1989
12. Rose SJ: Physical therapy diagnosis: Role and function. Phys Ther 69:535, 1989
13. Echternach JL, Rothstein JM: Hypothesis-oriented algorithms. Phys Ther 69: 559, 1989
14. O'Neill DL, Harris SR: Developing goals and objectives for handicapped children. Phys Ther 62:295, 1982
15. Zimmerman J: Goals and Objectives for Developing Normal Movement Patterns. Aspen, Rockville, MD, 1988
16. Bohannon RW: Objective measures. Phys Ther 69:80, 1989
17. Turek SL: Orthopaedics—Principles and Their Application. 4th Ed. Vol. 2. JB Lippincott, Philadelphia, 1984
18. Singleton MC, LeVeau BF: The hip joint: Structure, stability and stress. Phys Ther 55:957, 1975
19. Williams PL, Warwick R: Gray's Anatomy. 36th Ed. WB Saunders, Philadelphia, 1980
20. Maitland GD: The Vertebral Column—Examination and Recording Guide. Virgo Press, Adelaide, 1976
21. Van Hoesen LB: Passive movement in treatment of a painful hip. Bull Orthop Section APTA 2:9, 1977
22. Maitland GD: The hypothesis of adding compression when examining and treating synovial joints. J Orthop Sports Phys Ther 2:7, 1980

23. Wyke B: The neurology of joints: A review of general principles. Clin Rheum Dis 7:223, 1981
24. Crutchfield CA, Barnes MR: The Neurophysiologic Basis of Patient Treatment. Vol. III. Peripheral Components of Motor Control. Stokesville, Atlanta, 1984
25. Levi SJ, Maihafer GC: Traditional approaches to pain. p. 73. In Echternach JL (ed): Pain. Churchill Livingstone, New York, 1988
26. Henricson AS, Fredriksson K, Persson I, et al: The effect of heat and stretching on the range of hip motion. J Orthop Sports Phys Ther 6:110, 1984
27. Svarcova J, Trnavsky K, Zvarova J: The influence of ultrasound, galvanic current and shortwave diathermy on pain intensity in patients with osteoarthritis. Scand J Rheumatol Suppl 67:83, 1988
28. Mortiz U: Physical therapy and rehabilitation. Scand J Rheumatology Suppl 43: 49, 1982
29. Kowal MA: Review of physiological effects of cryotherapy. J Orthop Sports Phys Ther 5:66, 1983
30. Gersh MR, Wolf S: Applications of transcutaneous electrical nerve stimulation in the management of patients with pain—state of the art update. Phys Ther 65:314, 1985
31. Cailliet R: Soft Tissue Pain and Disability. FA Davis, Philadelphia, 1980
32. Grant R: Freud, joggers and strawberry pickers—entrapment neuropathies for all. p. 155. In Gilraine F, Sweeting L (eds): The Proceedings of the 5th International Conference of the International Federation of the Orthopaedic Manipulative Therapists, Whakatane, New Zealand, 1984
33. Roy S, Irvin R: Sports Medicine—Prevention, Evaluation, Management, and Rehabilitation. Prentice-Hall, Englewood Cliffs, NJ, 1983
34. Travell JG, Simons DG: Myofascial Pain and Dysfunction—The Trigger Point Manual. Williams & Wilkins, Baltimore, 1983
35. Simons DG: Myofascial pain syndromes. p. 209, 313. In Basmajian JV, Kirby RL (eds): Medical Rehabilitation. Williams & Wilkins, Baltimore, 1984
36. Halkovich LR, Personius WJ, Clamann HP, Newton RA: Effect of Fluorimethane[R] spray on passive hip flexion. Phys Ther 61:185, 1981
37. Newton RA: Effects of vapocoolants on passive hip flexion in healthy subjects. Phys Ther 65:1034, 1985
38. Barnes JF: Myofascial Release Seminar I. Pain and Stress Control Center, Paoli, PA, 1988
39. Mottice M, Goldberg D, Benner EK, Spoerl J: Soft Tissue Mobilization. JEMD Company, 1986
40. Crosman LJ, Chateauvert SR, Weisberg J: The effects of massage to the hamstring muscle group on range of motion. J Orthop Sport Phys Ther 6:168, 1984
41. Godges JJ, MacRae H, Longdon C, et al: The effects of two stretching procedures on hip range of motion and gait economy. J Orthop Sports Phys Ther 10:350, 1989
42. Sutton G: Hamstrung by hamstring strains: A review of the literature. J Orthop Sports Phys Ther 5:184, 1984
43. Stanton PE: Hamstring injuries in sprinting—the role of eccentric exercise. J Orthop Sports Phys Ther 10:343, 1989
44. Chamberlain G: Cyriax's friction massage: A review. J Orthop Sports Phys Ther 4:16, 1984
45. Rothstein JM: Muscle biology: Clinical considerations. Phys Ther 62:1823, 1982
46. Voss DE, Ionta MK, Myers BJ: Proprioceptive Neuromuscular Facilitation. 3rd Ed. Harper & Row, New York, 1985

47. Inman VT, Ralston HJ, Todd F: Human Walking. Williams & Wilkins, Baltimore, 1981
48. New York University Medical Center: Lower-Limb Orthotics. Postgraduate Medical School Prosthetics and Orthotics, New York, 1986
49. Lehmkuhl LD, Smith LK: Brunnstrom's Clinical Kinesiology. 4th Ed. FA Davis, Philadelphia, 1983
50. Feldenkrais M: Awareness through Movement. 2nd Ed. Harper & Row, New York, 1977
51. Kisner C, Colby LA: Therapeutic Exercise. Foundations and Techniques. FA Davis, Philadelphia, 1985
52. Mohr TM, Allison JD, Patterson R: Electromyographic analysis of the lower extremity during pedaling. J Orthop Sports Phys Ther 2:163, 1981
53. Hubley CL, Kozey JW, Stanish WD: The effects of static stretching exercises and stationary cycling on range of motion at the hip joint. J Orthop Sports Phys Ther 6:104, 1984
54. Negus RA, Rippe JM, Freedson P, Michaels J: Heart rate, blood pressure, and oxygen consumption during orthopaedic rehabilitation exercise. J Orthop Sports Phys Ther 8:346, 1987
55. Cooperman JM: Case studies: Isolated strain of the tensor fasciae latae. J Orthop Sports Phys Ther 5:201, 1984
56. Kornberg C, Lew P: The effect of stretching neural structures on grade one hamstring injuries. J Orthop Sports Phys Ther 10:481, 1989
57. Griffin J: Use of proprioceptive stimuli in therapeutic exercise. Phys Ther 54: 1072, 1974
58. Tanigawa M: Comparison of the hold-relax procedure and passive mobilization on increasing muscle length. Phys Ther 52:725, 1972
59. Markos PD: Ipsilateral and contralateral effects of proprioceptive neuromuscular facilitation techniques on hip motion and electromyographic activity. Phys Ther 59:1366, 1979
60. Bohannon RW: Effect of repeated eight-minute muscle loading on the angle of straight-leg-raising. Phys Ther 64:491, 1984
61. Thomas GJ: Swimming—an alternative form of therapy. Clin Management 9: 25, 1989
62. Mennet P, Egger B: Hüftdisziplin. Solbadklinik Rheinfelden, Rheinfelden, Switzerland, 1986
63. Paeth B: Schwimmtherapie 'Halliwick-Methode' nach James McMillan bei erwachsenenpatienten mit neurologischen erkrankungen. Z Krankengymnastik 36:100, 1984
64. Boyle AM: The Bad Ragaz ring method. Physiotherapy 67:265, 1981
65. Carr JH, Shepherd RB: A Motor Relearning Programme for Stroke. Aspen, Rockville, MD, 1987
66. Yamomoto S, Suto Y, Kawamura H, et al: Quantitative gait evaluation of hip diseases using principal component analysis. J Biomech 16:717, 1983
67. Neumann DA, Cook TM: Effect of load and carrying position on the electromyographic activity of the gluteus medius muscle during walking. Phys Ther 65:305, 1985
68. Clark JM, Haynor DR: Anatomy of the abductor muscles of the hip as studied by computed tomography. J Bone Joint Surg 69A:1021, 1987
69. Isacson J, Brostrom LA: Gait in rheumatoid arthritis: An electomyographic investigation. J Biomech 21:451, 1988

70. Neumann DA, Soderberg GL, Cook TM: Electromyographic analysis of hip abductor musculature in healthy right-handed persons. Phys Ther 69:431, 1989
71. Ely DD, Smidt GL: Effect of cane on variables of gait for patients with hip disorders. Phys Ther 57:507, 1977
72. Gogia PP, Braatz JH: Validity and reliability of leg length measurements. J Orthop Sports Phys Ther 8:185, 1986
73. Bandy WD, Sinning WE: Kinematic effects of heel lift use to correct lower limb length. J Orthop Sports Phys Ther 7:173, 1986
74. Andriacchi TP, Andersson GBJ, Fermier RW, et al: A study of lower-limb mechanics during stair climbing. J Bone Joint Surg 62A:749, 1980
75. Gore TA, Higginson GR, Stevens J: The kinematics of hip joints: Normal functioning. Clin Phys Physiol Meas 5:233, 1984
76. Brandstater ME: Activities of daily living. p. 246. In Basmajian JV, Kirby RL (eds): Medical Rehabilitation. Williams & Wilkins, Baltimore, 1984

APPENDIX 7-1

Exercises Following Manipulation of the Hip Under Anesthetic: Patient Instruction Sheet[a]

Lying on back (legs straight)
  1. Bend knee of affected leg as far as possible onto chest. Keep other leg flat on bed. Assist moving leg with hands.
  2. Keeping the knees straight and toes toward ceiling, move the affected leg away from other leg. Do *NOT* move the leg not being exercised.
  3. Slightly separate the legs. Roll legs in and out. Keep knees straight and hips on the bed.
  4. Lift leg with straight knee.

Lying on stomach
  5. Raise affected leg from the bed. Keep knee straight and do *NOT* roll pelvis in an effort to increase range of movement.

Standing (hold the back of a chair for support, keep body still when performing these exercises)
  6. Lift affected leg sideways, keeping knee straight and toes forward.
  7. Lift affected leg backwards, keeping knee straight and toes forward.

---

[a] Exercises are usually started the first day following manipulation. (From D. Yarreu, superintendent physiotherapist, Princess Elizabeth Orthopaedic Hospital, Exeter, England, with permission.)

Walking

8. Walk as able, even if only able to manage a short distance frequently. If you use a walking stick, this should be in the hand opposite the affected hip.

Stairs

9. Do stairs as a normal part of your day, if they can be done safely.

APPENDIX 7-2

McMillan's 10-Point Program: Pool Therapy

Program Steps	Treatment Activities
1. Mental adjustment—the patient gets used to the water	The patient is taken into the water and held at the thorax or pelvis by the therapist (if patient is fearful). Use activities that get the patient into deeper water. Begin practice breathing in the water.
2. Disengagement	The therapist moves away from the patient.
3. Vertical rotation control	The patient learns to move in an anteroposterior direction. All exercises begin in the sitting position, and the patient then starts to move anteriorly and posteriorly with feet still on the bottom of the pool. Also work on stabilization and maintenance of the sitting position by trying to disturb the patient's balance by touching him. Progress to pushing the patient off balance for anteroposterior balance recovery.

4. Lateral rotation control

The patient learns to move around his own body axis. Begin in supine float with arms abducted 90°. Move the pelvis in rotary motions to elicit equilibrium reactions. Change arms to adducted by side or overhead position and repeat. Therapist then changes hand placement to a point more distal than the pelvis. Patient lifts individual body segments out of the water.

5. Combined rotation control

Vertical and lateral rotation control are combined. Begin in sitting and disturb patient's balance in diagonals. With patient in supine, drag him through the water using rotary movement to simulate the feeling of combined rotation (lateral and vertical).

6. Mental inversion

The patient learns about buoyancy. Use underwater activities. Hold breath and sink to the bottom, so patient learns of buoyancy rather than the idea that water only pulls him down.

7. Balance is stillness

Patient learns to float and learns that to regain balance he must be still (no movement).

8. Turbulence gliding

The patient learns to glide by pushing off the side or bottom of pool, or the therapist pulls the patient and then lets go.

9. Simple progression

Progression from glide—patient uses hands and feet to progress.

10. Basic movement

The patient learns the first swim stroke— usually the back stroke.

Note: Treatment considerations:
   1. Which rotational control will be the most difficult?
   2. Which position will be used mainly in treatment—supine or sitting?
   3. Which technique will be most appropriate for use to meet the patient's goal?

The techniques are hierarchial, but steps can be skipped. The patient is NOT considered to be independent in the water, however, unless all 10 points of the program have been achieved.

(From C. Rodemers, P.T., Medizinisches Zentrum, Bad Ragaz, Switzerland with permission.)
(Adapted and modified from the program described by Paeth.[63])

8 | Athletic Injuries to the Hip

Susan D. Lambert

As larger numbers of people participate in athletic events, the care of athletic injuries assumes increasing importance. The evidence for this increasing importance can be seen in the number of clinics devoted to sports injuries as well as the increasing numbers of health professionals (physicians, physical therapists, athletic trainers) who are concerned with the care of these injuries. Not only are there increasing numbers of individuals of all ages actively engaged in sports activities, but the opportunity for sports activities has also increased. The variety of athletic activities that individuals can engage in throughout their entire life seems to have expanded enormously over the past several decades. Because of this, a chapter covering sports injuries to the hip and surrounding area is relevant to this text.

AVULSIONS

Apophyseal avulsions of the pelvis and proximal femur occur most commonly to male athletes 10 to 20 years old. This injury can occur at the area of the anterior iliac spine, especially during the middle to late teenage years, when the iliac crest unites with the ilium. Avulsions are generally a direct result of vigorous or uncoordinated activity, particularly forceful muscular contractions of the sartorius or tensor fasciae latae not counterbalanced by cocontracting agonists. Sports that require springing, kicking, running, and jumping can create this situation, and it is seen in activities such as sprinting, hurdling, pole-vaulting, high jumping, and punting.[1]

The accompanying pain is usually acute at onset and may continue for several weeks. While some athletes may be able to continue normal levels of activity, hip motion is often limited owing to pain and/or muscle spasm. Physical examination may reveal point tenderness, crepitus, and/or hematoma. A bony fragment may be palpable one inch or more below the anterior superior iliac spine. Active hip flexion or passive hip flexion with the hip beginning in extension will increase pain at this site.[2]

Prognosis for well-healing avulsion fractures is excellent, but a fibrous union may require surgical excision.[3] Proper treatment is conservative medical management, including transportation from injury site by stretcher with the hip and knee flexed. Ice and hip spica compression is the appropriate first aid, followed by bed rest, aspirin, and crutch ambulation with activity modification. Sitting is allowed with the hips slightly abducted.

Some exostosis or bony deformity may be persistently visible on radiographs. Athletes may return to normal activity following adequate rehabilitation for the return of strength, flexibility, and functional capacity. Whirlpool and moist heat may be of benefit during the initial stages of recovery.

Avulsion injuries may be prevented with careful physical screening and functional testing measures done before athletic participation. As muscular imbalances and discrepancies are noted, young athletes can be placed on appropriate exercise programs.

FRACTURES

Stress Fractures

Stress fractures most often occur in runners near the pubic symphysis or at the femoral neck region. Chronic, nonspecific tenderness in soft tissue of the inguinal area may exist with pain during extremes of hip motion. Symptoms usually occur following a long run. Diagnosis should be confirmed by radiography and/or bone scan during the early stages.[4,5]

Treatment includes rest and abstinence from athletic activity for 5 to 8 weeks, or until there is no hip pain at rest. The athlete may then progress from partial to full weightbearing with crutches, and from crutches to a cane as pain levels allow. When the individual is pain-free without assistive devices, swimming, biking, and walking may be done in quarter-mile increments. Progression of this program should be monitored based on pain. The athlete who begins to feel discomfort should be instructed to rest for 2 days and then resume the last level of pain-free activity. When the athlete can walk one mile pain-free and radiographs indicate that the site is well healed, previous activity levels may slowly be resumed.[6]

More severe cases of femoral neck stress fractures may require surgical intervention. Rehabilitation then may be more lengthy but will still utilize the same staged progression of activity discussed above. This injury can be prevented by progressive and gradual increases in workout distance and intensity.[7]

Fracture of Femoral Neck and Proximal Femoral Shaft

The usual cause of these injuries is a fall and a direct blow to the hip. The foot is planted and the hip is twisted. Skating and skiing are two activities where this type of fracture might present itself. Deformity exists in which the injured lower extremity is shortened and twisted outward. Fractures are often open, and there is significant blood loss. First aid requirements are as follows: (1) prevent hypovolemic shock; (2) sterile pressure dressing to open areas; (3) check skin color, temperature, and pulse of foot for possible vascular injury; (4) traction, realignment, and splinting by trained medical personnel.[5,6]

Ilium Wing Fractures

The mechanism of injury is usually a direct blow, such as that sustained from a fall (e.g., as in horseback riding). There is extreme tenderness along the iliac crest and down the wing of the ilium. Often secondary spasm of the abdominal muscles causes further pain. Anterior-posterior radiographs of the ilium are most effective in determining a definitive diagnosis.[3]

Treatment of Fractures

Subacute treatment begins with complete bed rest and casting from the lower costal area to just above the knee. A corset or taping may be adequate if the fragment is not severely displaced. Healing time is approximately 6 to 8 weeks with ambulation as discomfort permits.[3]

CONTUSIONS
Hip Pointer

Probably the most widely discussed and feared contusion of the hip region is that of injury to the iliac crest. Commonly referred to as a hip pointer, a contusion occurs by direct blow, usually at or near the anterior superior iliac spine. Often there is accompanying bleeding, edema, and pain with palpation, active trunk movement, coughing, laughing, or sneezing. Avulsion of the external obliques is a frequent secondary problem.

Treatment consists of ice and anti-inflammatory medication during the first 48 to 72 hours postinjury, with gentle, graded stretching as symptoms subside. Transcutaneous electrical nerve stimulation (TENS) may be beneficial to those athletes whose competition schedules do not allow a longer rest period.[8]

Preventing this injury or protecting it from further trauma requires adequate padding of the iliac crest. This may be accomplished with a wide variety of materials, such as a high-density foam/orthoplast/moleskin fabrication or modification of football hip pad (Fig. 8-1). These may be secured by strapping the pad

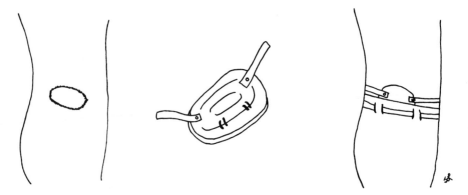

Fig. 8-1. Protection for hip pointer. **(A)** After marking tender area of body with felt tip pen, press foam, felt, or moleskin against marked area and cut padding where pen marks indicate. **(B)** Mark orthoplast in same shape and size as padding. After heating, mold orthoplast in a cup-like shape then cut belt loop holes and attach padding to concave side. **(C)** Attach measured waist strap to orthoplast using football shoulder pad strapping and helmet snaps and screws. Strap pad in place, then thread pant belt through pants and pad. (Based on information in Gallaspy.[10]).

through the uniform pant belt loop from inside or by sewing a pad-holding pocket inside the uniform pant.[9,10] Additional support can be obtained through the recommended taping technique shown in Figure 8-2.[11]

Sacroiliac Joint Contusion

It is well known that sacral pads are required for most contact sports. This area is highly vulnerable to contusion when not sufficiently padded. Tenderness following trauma here can be diffuse or sharply localized to the sacrum and/or iliac spines. Possible fractures should be ruled out by radiography.

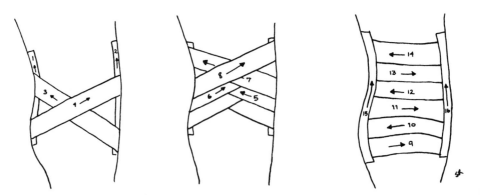

Fig. 8-2. Taping technique for hip pointer. This may be enclosed with an Ace compression wrap.

Initial treatment is the immediate application of cold and compression, best accomplished through the use of an ice pack and elastic sacroiliac support. Following the 48 to 72 hour acute phase, heat may be applied and gentle exercise begun. William's flexion exercises are particularly helpful in increasing sacroiliac joint mobility and decreasing pain. While this contusion is painful, it is not terribly disabling. An athlete may, therefore, resume play when pain-free and fully mobile, providing proper padding is utilized.[3]

Coccygeal Contusion

Coccyx injury is most likely to occur from a fall onto a hard surface into the sitting position. Ice and roller skaters are susceptible candidates, although it has been known to happen following a lay-up on the basketball court, a high forceful kick on the soccer field, or an inadvertent blow from another player's shoe. Fracture can also result; however, no immobilization is necessary other than the use of a girdle and padding to the coccyx for sport participation.[3]

Standard first aid procedures of rest, ice, and compression during the initial 3 days postinjury are recommended. Heat may then be useful to help reduce pain until the player feels ready to return to practice and competition, usually within 2 to 3 weeks. It should be emphasized that athletes recovering from coccygeal injuries need to maintain cardiovascular endurance and upper body strength through activities such as swimming and progressive resistive exercise in supine and prone positions, but they should avoid the painful position of sitting.

Contusion Injuries to the Groin

While damage to the pubic symphysis during athletics is rare, contusion to the mons pubis in female equestrians and gymnasts is fairly common. Hematomas usually develop rapidly and the area becomes tender upon palpation. Aspiration is not generally recommended or successful owing to the infiltration of blood into the fat pad. Standard first aid and treatment techniques for superficial hematoma are advised.[3]

The testicles are often a site of painful contusion for male athletes, despite their relatively protected location between the thighs. Mechanism of injury is almost always inadvertent during activities such as football tackles. Symptoms include excruciating local pain and nausea. There may be muscle spasm, hemorrhage, and fluid effusion, all dependent on the intensity of the impact. Generally, there are no secondary complications; however, the sports therapist should seek additional medical attention if spermatic cord torsion is suspected. This twisting of the testicles within the scrotal sac produces pain, nausea, vomiting, and inflammation, not relieved by ice and techniques to reduce muscle spasm. Additional signs include evidence of swollen veins within the testicle and a heavy feeling of the scrotum. Atrophy of the testicle occurs if medical treatment is not obtained. Traumatic hydrocele, or excess fluid accumulation in the tunica vaginalis, is also a secondary complication, requiring a physician referral.[11]

When simple contusion of the testicles is suspected, however, either of two highly effective techniques may be employed for immediate relief:

1. Active-assistive hip flexion in the supine position followed by local application of ice pack is effective (Fig. 8-3).

2. Position athlete in long-sit position with arms folded across the chest. The therapist grasps the torso from behind by locking his or her arms under the arms and around the chest of the athlete. The athlete is then lifted several inches off the ground with a quick drop to the ground following. The mild jolt is thought to "short circuit" the pain impulses from the testicles (Fig. 8-4). As in the first technique, ice packs should follow immediately and continue for at least 24 hours, 15 minutes on, 1 hour off. After the acute stage, moist heat packs, whirlpool, and sitz baths are helpful.[11]

Overall, the male genitalia can be effectively protected in many sports through the use of the athletic supporter and/or cup.[7] The young male athlete may require reminding, as these devices are sometimes regarded as uncomforta-

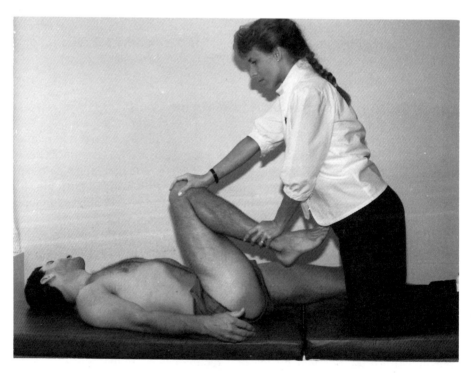

Fig. 8-3.   Treatment technique for testicular spasm includes active-assistive hip flexion, followed by ice pack.

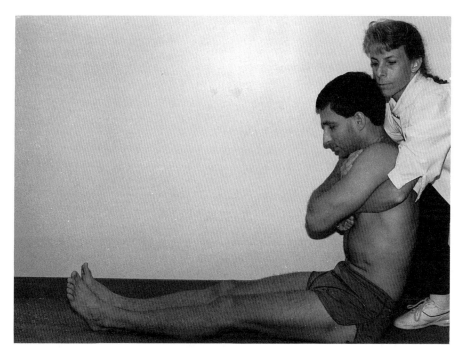

Fig. 8-4. Alternate treatment technique for testicular spasm. This technique should not be performed on any athlete suspected of hip joint, sacroiliac, or lumbosacral dysfunction.

ble, unnecessary, or embarrassing. Education by the coach, therapist, and parents is helpful for compliance. Also, a well-trained athlete has been taught the response of quick thigh and trunk flexion to further protect this area from oncoming, potentially injurious forces.[3]

SPRAINS

Hip Joint Sprains

The classic history given by the sufferer of hip joint sprain is rigorous twisting of the lower extremity or twisting of the trunk while the lower extremity is firmly planted. The mechanism of injury can occur as an active movement by the athlete or can be due to external impacting forces. Upon examination, the athlete will usually be unable to circumduct the leg owing to pain.[11] Treatment includes an iced Ace wrap hip spica (Fig. 8-5) and crutches for partial weight-bearing ambulation. Crutch walking should continue until the athlete can achieve pain-free gait.[5] Strength should be restored to equal that of the uninvolved hip, using progressive resistive exercise techniques. Functional tests

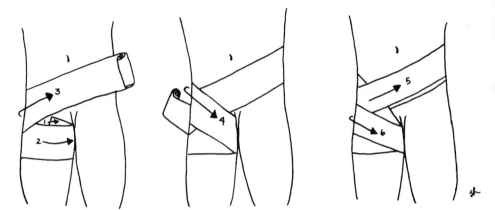

Fig. 8-5. Hip spica Ace wrapping technique for trauma to the hip. This is a highly effective first aid technique when the Ace wrap has been wetted and then placed in the freezer. Direction of wrapping may be reversed for injuries to the outer hip and buttock.

such as hopping, sprinting, backwards running, cutting, and pivoting must all be satisfactorily passed (no pain, no limp, no alteration in skill performance) prior to the athlete's return to play.

Sacroiliac Joint Sprains

The ligaments of the sacroiliac joints are so strong that one should be very cautious about using the term sacroiliac sprain. This injury is rare in young athletes. More common is the problem of inflammation of the sacroiliac joint, which is discussed later in this chapter. In ruling out a true sacroiliac joint sprain, the sports therapist should not forget to include the sacroiliac compression and distraction tests as well as the Fabere (Patrick's) test (Fig. 8-6).

Sprain of the Ligaments of the Pubic Symphysis

Forceful bilateral hip abduction can cause a sprain of the pubic symphysis ligaments in the adolescent athlete, as the symphysis is not yet firmly fixed. The pelvic ring can be compressed by circumferential taping or the use of a long fitted lumbosacral support. This initial treatment (along with rest and anti-inflammatory agents) is followed by the application of heat after the first 48 to 72 hours postinjury. Healing may take many weeks; therefore, horseback riding, skiing, and specific activities such as straddle vaulting, splits, and straddle moves on the uneven parallel bars in gymnastics must be temporarily avoided. The prognosis is positive provided that appropriate diagnosis and treatment are made.[3]

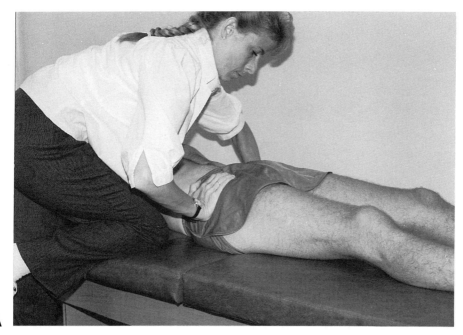

A

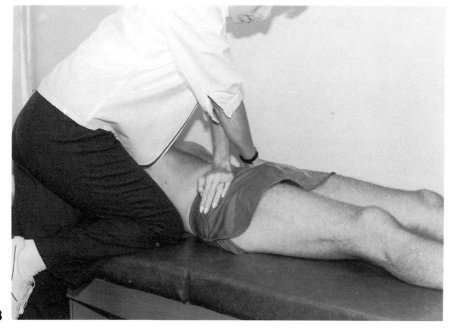

B

Fig. 8-6. (**A**) Passive sacroiliac joint compression. (**B**) Passive sacroiliac joint distraction. (*Figure continues.*)

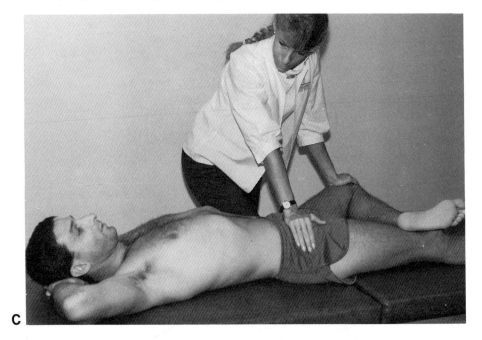

C

Fig. 8-6 (*Continued*).   (**C**) Passive flexion-abduction-external rotation (Fabere) for Patrick's test. Do these tests exacerbate symptoms, relieve discomfort, or make no change?

MUSCLE STRAINS
Adductor Strains

The hip adductor muscles (gracilis, pectineus, and adductors longus, brevis, and magnus) are the most frequently strained muscle complex of the groin region. Jumping, running, or twisting are suspect in the cause of this injury, particularly when external rotation of the affected leg is an added component of the activity.[11] In addition, the adductor group can be strained from an activity such as a forceful soccer kick that is stopped by an opponent's foot, or by a sliding tackle with an abducted leg. The signs and symptoms are easily recognizable:[12]

1.   Twinging or stabbing pain in the groin area with quick starts and stops
2.   Edema or echemosis several days postinjury
3.   Pain with manual resistance to adduction
4.   Possibly a palpable defect and bony tenderness in severe ruptures
5.   Muscle guarding
6.   Pseudoparalysis or false paralysis of the extremity resulting from pain and muscle guarding

In cases of severe rupture, radiographs are needed to rule out avulsion. Proper treatment is critical, both in the acute and subacute phases of healing, as a "groin pull" can easily become a troublesome, chronic and reoccurring problem. Initial treatment includes rest, intermittent iced hip spica compression, and elevation. Anti-inflammatory agents are also effective. Crutch walking is recommended until acute groin pain subsides. Whirlpool, ultrasound, and a graded range of motion program should follow. When the athlete can obtain full pain-free movement, progressive resistive exercise is begun until equal strength with the contralateral hip is acquired. Continuation of hip spica compression and the use of TENS may be helpful.[5] Functional relationships between ipsilateral muscle groups should also be evaluated for possible predisposing muscle strength imbalances. Ideally, these imbalances should be discovered by preseason physical examinations to identify those athletes at high risk for strains to the hip region.[12]

Iliopsoas Strain

As the strongest flexor of the hip joint, the iliopsoas is also one of the more frequently strained muscles of this area.[6] Mechanism of injury is forced extension of the lower extremity while the hip is actively flexed (e.g., quick starts in running). The athlete will typically hold the guarding hip and thigh in a relaxed position of flexion, adduction, and external rotation. Manual resistance against this position increases discomfort, as does attempts at acceleration and high-stepping activity. Following this injury, the athlete (in frustration) is usually physically required to discontinue participation. Recovery can be lengthy, and a premature decision to return to play only recreates the above scenario.[3]

Radiography following this injury is of the utmost importance in the adolescent athlete, owing to increased danger of avulsion of the epiphyseal site located here. Fibrous union is the usual natural healing method; therefore, surgery is rarely indicated. Treatment, as with all strains, begins with rest, ice, and compression. As symptoms subside, hip extension should be encouraged to prevent flexion contracture formation. The athlete can be instructed to sleep in the prone position, which will assist this effort. Heat and a graded resistive exercise program are indicated during the following weeks, with the use of a heat-retaining compression garment to aid in pain-free activity.[3] Proper warm-up and cool-down are critical after this injury, giving specific attention to functional training for optimum use of this muscle.

Rectus Abdominis Strain

Strain of the rectus abdominis may occur at its attachment to the pubis, along the inner end of Poupart's ligament.[3] The movements and activities in sports such as tennis, weight lifting, gymnastics, rowing, and wrestling are often the cause. Pole-vaulters, javelin throwers, and shot-putters are at risk for this injury if they do not have adequate abdominal strength or use proper technique. Rectus abdominis strain usually occurs when the muscle is strongly contracting while it is quickly moved into a stretched and elongated position. It may be difficult to differentiate this condition from inflammation of the internal abdominal organs, such as the appendix, and therefore, the athlete should be examined by a physician when any doubt exists.[6]

Mild strains may only take several weeks to heal. Premature return to play can create large muscle ruptures, leading to hernia formation in the abdominal wall. This problem is discussed in further detail later in this chapter. Initial treatment is that of all muscle strains—rest, ice, compression, and anti-inflammatory agents. Heat, gentle stretching, and gradual progressive resistive exercise are helpful in the later stages. Training and retraining of the rectus abdominis should include half sit-ups, done slowly with bent knees, to eliminate compensation by the iliopsoas.[6]

Gluteus Medius Strain

Strain of the gluteus medius is usually an overuse syndrome, chronic in origin and often seen in long-distance runners. A contributing factor may be due to overload caused by weakness in surrounding muscles. Pain occurs over the trochanteric region with active contraction against resistance. If there is palpable tenderness while the athlete is relaxed and if active movement is pain-free, one should consider that the condition is a possible trochanteric bursitis. Avulsion of the greater trochanteric epiphysis of the adolescent athlete must also be ruled out. Heat modalities are the treatments of choice, preferably ultrasound or diathermy, owing to the depth of this thick, dense muscle. Attention should be directed to the examination of strength in all hip extensors and external rotator muscles with regard to prevention and rehabilitation.[8,11]

Hamstring Strain

Perhaps the most dreaded muscular strain by the athlete is that of the hamstring muscle group. The list of potential causes of this injury is long; poor posture, decreased flexibility, inappropriate quadricep/hamstring strength ratios, comparative bilateral strength deficits, lack of coordination, and fatigue have all been cited as causes.[5]

One can usually get a clear history of the development of this condition because the athlete will report that immediate pain was felt during full-stride running or while quickly decelerating. On examination there is tenderness, especially during stretch of the hamstrings, and in severe cases, ecchymosis, hemorrhage, and a muscle defect may be visible several days postinjury. Crutches may be necessary for ambulation.[5]

After acute-stage treatment of ice, rest, and compression, it is imperative to minimize the consequences of inelastic scar tissue formation within the muscle belly. Improper management can lead to recurrent tears and a condition known as the hamstring syndrome, to be discussed later in this chapter. Scar massage, gentle stretching, and phonophoresis can be initiated early to reduce the risk of this occurrence. A felt or foam pad over the injury site, held in place by an Ace wrap or neoprene sleeve, is often helpful in decreasing pain by warmth and compression.[12]

All preseason evaluations and hamstring rehabilitation programs should include testing and training for appropriate quadricep/hamstring ratios as well as bilateral equality of strength. The importance of flexibility must be emphasized, and athletes should be educated in proper warm-up and cool-down techniques.[12] Ideally, warming up includes moves that mimic the actual event to be executed, but started at the 50 to 75 percent level of effort with gradual increases in intensity building to 100 percent or maximal effort. This technique can be easily visualized by picturing a low, slow-motion karate kick, with progression to a fast, high kick above waist level. The cool-down should reverse this technique to bring the athlete from high levels of energy expenditure back to slower resting levels. Cool-down is an especially important time to work on flexibility, when muscles are warm and relaxed. Static stretching is the method of choice for hamstring stretching, as well as for all muscle groups. Proper form is demonstrated in Figure 8-7. The contralateral extremity is bent inward, to reduce stress

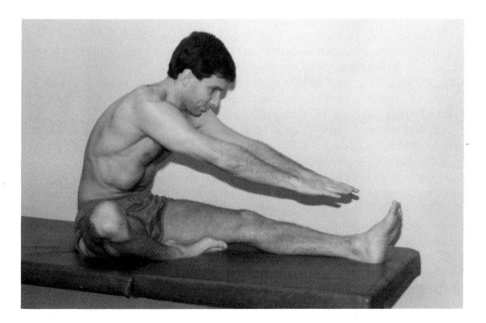

Fig. 8-7.   Proper form for passive stretching of the hamstrings.

on the medial structures of the knee. The stretch should be maintained for a minimum of 20 seconds before advancing further.

Rehabilitation time of hamstring strains varies considerably—2 to 3 weeks for mild injuries; 2 to 6 months for severe conditions. In any case, because of the frequent reoccurrence of hamstring pulls, an athlete should not be permitted to return to full participation until flexibility, strength, and appropriate muscular balances have been restored.[5]

INFLAMMATORY CONDITIONS

Synovitis

This inflammation of the tissues surrounding the hip joint can be the result of joint sprain or direct trauma. Any hip motion may cause a generalized soreness. In addition, the athlete is likely to be point tender with palpation of the greater trochanter. Synovitis of the hip joint is seen in children below the age of 10. Symptoms can often be similar to more serious disease processes such as osteomyelitis, tuberculosis, tumors, and rheumatic disorders. It is therefore imperative that young athletes with these signs and symptoms be examined by a physician.[6] Synovitis responds well to daily heat applications. As pain is relieved, normal hip movement and gait patterns are restored.[11]

Trochanteric Bursitis and the Snapping Hip

The snapping hip can be seen in gymnasts, dancers, and runners who have created an imbalance in the hip musculature from repetitive flexion with external rotation of the hip. As the joint capsule and ligaments also become less stable, an audible and palpable snapping occurs on movement. Pain within the tensor fasciae latae and trochanteric bursa subsequently occurs.[11]

Initial treatment should focus on reducing spasm of the tensor fasciae latae and inflammation of the bursa. Rest and phonophoresis followed by ice massage is an excellent means of providing prompt relief. Oral or injected anti-inflammatory drugs may also be effective. Chronic conditions can be surgically corrected by removing the bursa and releasing tension on the tensor fasciae latae muscle, although this is rarely necessary.[8]

Reconditioning and prevention should concentrate on flexibility of soft tissues and strength balance among the hip's surrounding muscles. Gait and postural evaluation are very useful in determining who is predisposed to this condition. Important findings might include leg length discrepancies or alignment problems.[8] The female athlete generally has a wider pelvis and more prominent trochanters and the tensor may bow at a more acute angle than in the male.[3] This may explain the frequency with which this problem occurs in women.

Osteitis Pubis

As long-distance running has gained in popularity, osteitis pubis has become a more common problem. This condition is also seen in soccer, football, and wrestling athletes.[11] This chronic inflammatory condition is caused by stress placed on the pubic symphysis from the overexertion of muscles in this area. Symptoms include groin pain, which may radiate toward the lower abdomen or the inner thigh. There may be point tenderness over the pubic tubercle, and the adductor muscles may be in spasm. When the condition is severe, the athlete may even exhibit a waddling gait.[8]

Treatment includes rest, ice and anti-inflammatory agents initially, followed by heat modalities.[6] A slow and progressive strengthening program should begin after acute symptoms are abated, including work for the abdominal, groin, adductor, and lower back musculature.[8]

Sacroiliac Inflammation and Dysfunction

Sacroiliitis is often revealed during winter sport activities and more often in male than female athletes, ages 15 to 35 years. Discomfort is almost always worse in the morning and following periods of inactivity.[6] Careful history may trace the problem back to incidents such as a change in shoes, running terrain, or training exercises. Even seemingly trivial events like stepping in a pothole can create the onset of sacroiliac inflammation and dysfunction. Running in popular long-distance races where roadways are crowded with participants can lead to improper running technique. Thus, this disorder is not solely limited to the untrained athlete. When running form is compromised, either by ignorance or circumstance, the result may create abnormal pelvic rotation. In sacroiliac dysfunction, the ilium will often wedge and lock on the sacrum, resulting in pain and inflammation.[13]

Examination for this condition should include orthopaedic and neurologic testing to rule out lumbar spine pathology. A complete postural assessment is also critical. Ankylosing spondylitis, psoriatic arthritis, Reiter's syndrome, and reactive arthritis have been associated with inflammation of the sacroiliac joints. Radiographs, computed tomography, magnetic imagery, and blood and electrolyte studies may be helpful in ruling out these conditions.[14]

When all associated areas provide negative findings, three specific orthopaedic tests should be employed, as described by Whieldon and Winiewicz[13]: standing flexion, sitting flexion, and long sitting (Fig. 8-8). Muscle energy techniques as described by Erhard and Bowling[15] prove highly successful in unlocking the sacroiliac joint and restoring normal movement (Fig. 8-9). Standard modalities of heat, ice, and electrical stimulation may provide temporary relief. Anti-inflammatory agents may smooth locally irritated soft tissue structures. Prevention lies in the removal of the cause of the problem, that is, change in running technique, terrain, or shoes.

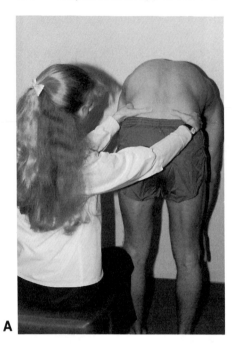
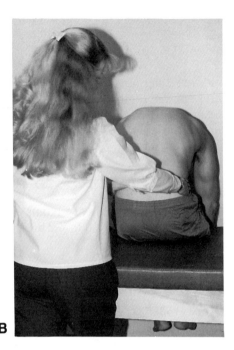
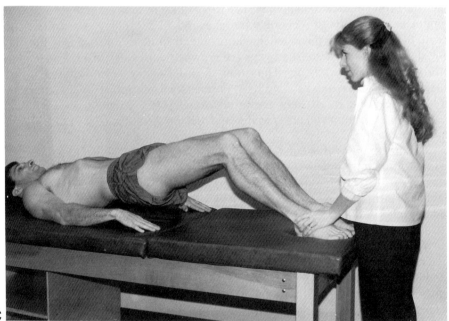

Fig. 8-8. (**A**) Active standing flexion test. (**B**) Active sitting flexion test. Observe the movement of the posterior superior iliac spines (PSIS). The cranially moving PSIS is the involved side. A sacrum and ilium moving as one unit creates a blocked sacroiliac (S-I) joint. (**C**) Bridging to relax and prepare hip musculature for the active long sitting test. (*Figure continues.*)

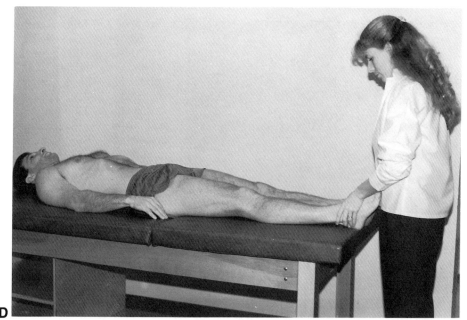

D

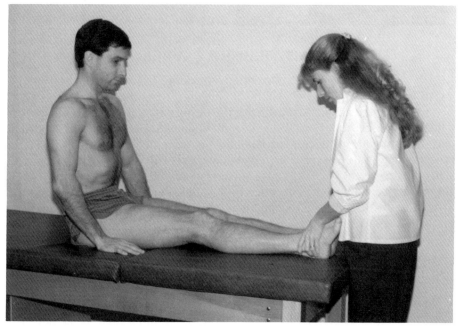

E

Fig. 8-8 (*Continued*).   (**D**) Visually measuring leg length and the position of the malleoli. (**E**) Athlete actively rising to the long-sit position; leg length and malleolus positions reevaluated for changes. The posterior ilium: Acetabulum is superior and ventral. Involved leg is short in supine and long in long sitting. The anterior ilium: Acetabulum is inferior and dorsal. Involved leg is long in supine and short in long sitting.

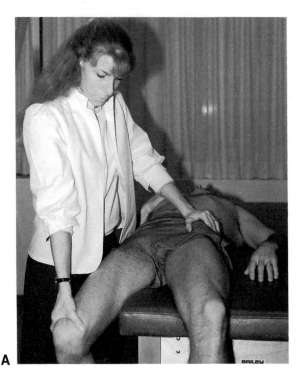

A

Fig. 8-9. (**A**) Muscle energy correction technique for the posterior ilium. Stand on involved side, stabilize noninvolved hip with hand most cephalad to athlete. Passively flex involved hip and knee fully. Athlete actively flexes involved hip (3 to 5 seconds) against therapist's unyielding hand. Upon relaxation, involved leg is gently pressed into further extension. Repeat full procedure four to six times. Reevaluate clinical signs.[16] (*Figure continues.*)

NERVE ENTRAPMENT SYNDROME

Piriformis Syndrome

Owing to the anatomic location of the piriformis, spasm of this muscle can compress the sciatic nerve, producing radiating sciaticalike pain. This syndrome may develop due to decreased flexibility or repetitive, vigorous use of the posterior hip musculature. Evaluation reveals positive Pace's and Freiberg's signs.[16] Treatment best suited for this condition includes gentle, static stretching, ice massaging, and coolant spray and stretch techniques (Fig. 8-10).[8] Stretching before and after athletic activity should be continued as a preventative measure.

Hamstring Syndrome

Recurrent hamstring strains or excessive overstretching of the hamstrings can lead to entrapment of the sciatic nerve. Symptoms present as pain with sitting, with stretching of the affected muscles, and during sprinting and hurdling activities. The athlete may describe the pain as sciaticlike sensations from the area of the lower buttock into the posterior thigh.

Myelograms, computed tomography, and magnetic resonance imagery will help rule out a lumbar spine cause of this radiating pain. Physical therapy

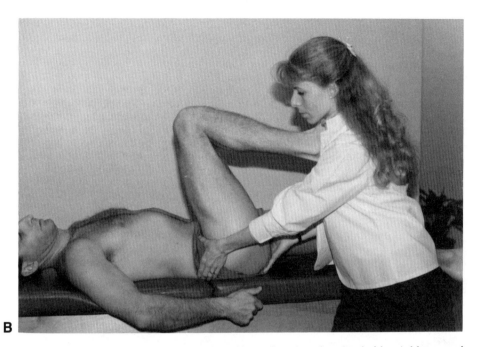

(B) Muscle energy technique for anterior ilium. Stand on involved side. Athlete maximally actively flexes hip and knee on the involved side. Hand placement for therapist is under the ischial tuberosity and over the anterior iliac spine (ASIS) of the involved side. With the athlete's foot on the therapist's chest, the leg is passively flexed. The athlete then produces an isometric contraction against the therapist (3 to 5 seconds). Further passive flexion is then applied by the therapist, using the hands to assist the hip into a pelvic tilt. Repeat full technique four to five times. Reevaluate for changes in clinical signs. (Based on information in Gallaspy.[10]).

modalities may fail to give more than very short-term relief to these patients. Surgical intervention is a relatively simple procedure and provides good results. The operative technique involves the sectioning of two to three tense, tendonlike bands that are typically found in the attachment of the biceps femoris, just anterior to the sciatic nerve. Athletic activity can be gradually resumed in the 3 to 6 weeks following surgery, with special attention given to proper muscle training.[16]

Meralgia Paresthetica

Meralgia paresthetica involves compression of the lateral femoral cutaneous nerve of the thigh. It can also occur to other nerves that traverse the hip, such as the ilioinguinal, genitofemoral, obturator, and anterior cutaneous nerves of the thigh. Compression evolves because of their anatomic locations about the groin and genital folds, along with secondary contributing factors of sudden

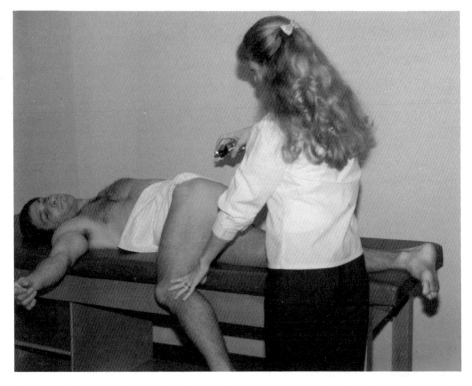

Fig. 8-10. Spray and stretch technique for the treatment of piriformis syndrome using Fluori-Methane coolant spray.

weight change, overstress on the abdominal muscles, or tight athletic undergarments or equipment.[6,17]

Signs and symptoms usually include pain (either local or radiating) and numbness with decreased sensation to light touch and pin prick testing. Treatment is concerned with eliminating the original cause and applying ice intermittently for 48 to 72 hours. Participation may be allowed within the athlete's pain tolerance. Local anesthetic injection or iontophoresis may reduce pain in more severe cases. Prevention of meralgia paresthetica and similar nerve entrapment syndromes requires proper fitting of athletic equipment and uniforms with regard to the athlete's weight, playing position, and exercise intensity.[17]

HERNIA

Herniation is the protrusion of underlying tissues through a weak section of muscle and peritoneum. Over 75 percent of all sports-related hernias are classified as inguinal, involving the inguinal canal area of the groin. They are most often seen in male athletes. Femoral hernias, on the other hand, are protrusions in the anterior proximal thigh region, just below the groin fold, and are more commonly seen in female athletes. Abdominal hernias are a third type, easily diagnosed by thermography, using a contrast medium to reveal an abnormal protrusion in the abdominal wall. Seen frequently in soccer players, abdominal hernias usually exist on the same side as the athlete's dominant kicking leg.[6]

History may reveal a past episode of contusion or strain to the area. Protrusion and pain may increase with coughing, sneezing, and strenuous exercise. Precautions should be taken to avoid further irritation by falls or blows. A complication known as strangulated hernia can occur in which the protruding sac's circulation is occluded. Gangrene and even death may follow if proper surgical attention is not sought. In the uncomplicated hernia, mild forms of exercise may be resumed 3 to 4 weeks postsurgery. Progressive resistive strength training may begin 2 to 2.5 months postoperatively.[11]

SUMMARY

In this chapter, the causes of the most common athletic injuries occurring in the hip and pelvic region were discussed. In addition, pertinent factors in the examination of these conditions were discussed and suggestions for the prevention of these injuries were made. Finally, a brief description of treatment methods and principles was offered to guide the therapist in this area of patient management.

Therapists treating those individuals who engage in athletic endeavors have enormous influence in their treatment programs and are in an ideal position to promote athletic injury prevention. Suggestions about warming up and cooling down, proper equipment, and technique are all important in managing these patients and support the role of the therapist in examination, assessment, and treatment of athletic injuries.

REFERENCES

1. Miller ML: Avulsion fractures of the anterior superior iliac spine in high school track. Athletic Training 17:57, 1982
2. Anderson JL, George F, Krakauer LJ, et al: 1982 Year Book of Sports Medicine. Year Book Medical Publishers, Chicago, 1982
3. O'Donohue DH: Treatment of Injuries to Athletes. 3rd Ed. WB Saunders, Philadelphia, 1976
4. Fullerton LR, Jr., Snowdy HA: Femoral neck stress fractures. Am J Sports Med 16:365, 1988
5. Ellison AE, Boland AL, Jr., DeHaven KE, et al (eds): Athletic Training and Sports Medicine. American Academy of Orthopaedic Surgery, Chicago, 1984
6. Peterson L, Renstrom P: Sports Injuries—Their Prevention and Treatment. Year Book Medical Publishers, Chicago, 1986
7. Morris AF: Sports Medicine Handbook. Wm. C. Brown Publishers, Dubuque, IA 1985
8. Roy S, Irvin R: Sports Medicine—Prevention, Evaluation, Management, and Rehabilitation. Prentice-Hall, Englewood Cliffs, NJ, 1983

9. Deutsch B, Fashouer T: Football hip pad protection for hip pointers and A-C sprains of ice hockey players. Athletic Training 16:238, 1981

10. Gallaspy JB, Maneval MW: Protective padding for a hip pointer. Athletic Training 21:128, 1986

11. Klafs CE, Arnheim DD: Modern Principles of Athletic Training. CV Mosby, St Louis, 1989

12. Casperson PC, Kaverman D (eds): Groin and hamstring injuries. Athletic Training 17:43, 1982

13. Whieldon TJ, Winiewicz TW: Sacroiliac dysfunction in runners. Athletic Training 21:15, 1986

14. American Health Consultants, Inc.: Inflammatory conditions can cause hip pain. Back Basics, October 1988

15. Erhard R, Bolwing R: The recognition and management of the pelvic component of lowback and sciatic pain. Bull Orthop Sect APTA 2:4, 1977

16. Puranen J, Orava S: The hamstring syndrome—a new diagnosis of gluteal sciatic pain. Am J Sports Med 16:517, 1988

17. Kolb JJ: Compression of the lateral femoral cutaneous nerve: Meralgia paresthetica. Athletic Training 18:304, 1983

9 | Role of the Hip in Posture and Gait

Carol A. Oatis

The purpose of this chapter is to discuss the behavior of the hip under the static conditions of quiet standing and during the dynamic conditions of locomotion. Much research has been done describing the kinematic (displacement history) and kinetic (force) parameters of the hip during function. More recently, investigators have examined controlling factors during various functional activities. In this chapter, I discuss the present understanding of the hip's function in quiet standing and during locomotion. The concepts include the traditional descriptive data of motion and force characteristics but also incorporate theories on how the hip joint controls and is controlled by other factors during these activities.

QUIET STANDING

Erect posture has been described by many as the correct alignment of several bony landmarks along a plumb line.[1-3] The alignment of the hip during standing is determined by the relative position of the pelvis on the femur. Kendall and McCreary[3] stated that normal anatomic variability of the pelvis precludes a standard for pelvic alignment with respect to the horizontal plane. Rather, they reported that one accepted norm for pelvic alignment is with respect to a vertical plane defining normal pelvic alignment as that in which the anterior superior iliac spines (ASIS) are in the same vertical plane as the pubic symphysis (Fig. 9-1). Harty[4] used a similar standard but reported that in females the ASIS may be up to 1 cm anterior to the pubic symphysis. The femur is approximately vertical, with the line of gravity passing through the greater

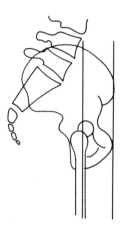

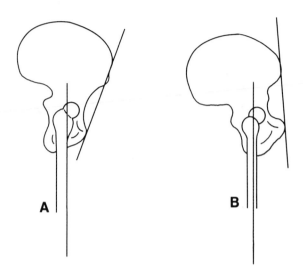

Fig. 9-1. ASIS and pubic symphysis are parallel to each other and femur is approximately parallel to both (ASIS and pubic symphysis).

Fig. 9-2. (**A**) Pelvis is in anterior pelvic tilt putting hip in relative position of flexion. (**B**) Pelvis is in posterior pelvic tilt putting hip in relative position of extension.

trochanter and just anterior to the lateral epicondyle.[3] In this position, the hip joint is approximately in neutral between flexion and extension. However, the exact position of the hip in normal posture continues to be debated. Soderberg[5] did state that it is doubtful that the hip is in maximum extension in erect posture. When the pelvis is rotated anteriorly the relative hip position is one of flexion, while conversely, a posterior pelvic tilt puts the hip in extension (Fig. 9-2). The presence of a hip flexion contracture has been associated with an anterior pelvic tilt, increased lumbar lordosis, and low back pain. However, Day et al.[6] found no statistical difference between the pelvic alignment in normal subjects and that in patients with chronic low back pain but did identify an increase in the hip flexion angle in quiet standing in patients with chronic low back pain. A possible explanation for this controversy is the difficulty of measuring pelvic alignment and thus the exact position of the hip.[7]

Control of the hip in the sagittal plane is reportedly provided by the iliopsoas muscle. Basmajian[8] stated that the line of gravity passes through the greater trochanter in quiet standing. Since the greater trochanter lies posterior to the hip joint, he anticipated that hip flexors would be required to maintain stability. Activity of the iliacus as shown by electromyography supports this theory. In addition, in the presence of hip flexor weakness as in paraplegia, patients find stability in standing by hyperextending the hip joint and apparently using the passive support of the anterior hip joint capsule and the ilio-, ischio-, and pubofemoral ligaments.[9]

Symmetry is purported to be an important criterion of normalcy in standing posture in the frontal plane. Yet, several researchers have suggested that asymmetry is not unusual among apparently normal subjects.[3,10,11] Kendall attributes the presence of asymmetry to asymmetric function resulting from hand dominance. The characteristic right-hand dominant posture described by Kendall and McCreary[3] consists, in part, of a lower right shoulder and an elevated pelvis on the right side. The resulting pelvic obliquity places the right hip in an adducted position and the left hip in an abducted position (Fig. 9-3). This pelvic alignment alters the resting length for a prolonged period and may result in strength changes in the muscle,[3,12] specifically weakness. This phenomenon has come to be known as stretch weakness. Kendall and McCreary[3] reported the presence of such weakness in the right hip abductors in right-handed people. However, Neumann et al.[10] failed to identify similar weakness in subjects with the right-handed posture. Neuman et al.[10] did note that differences in the slopes of the torque-angle curves of the left and right hips were consistent with the concepts of stretch weakness; that is, the slope was steeper for the right hip than for the left, showing that the abduction strength had a greater decrease in strength as the hip abduction angle increased. The prevalence of the right-handed posture as described by Kendall and McCreary[3] has not been determined, nor has a clear cause-effect relationship been established between this posture and hip abduction strength. In other words, it is not known whether asymmetric function results in muscle strength asymmetries that then cause asymmetric posture or whether the function causes uneven posture that then results in asymmetric strength. However, these data support the need for further investigation into the relationship between muscle strength and static posture at the hip. It also suggests to the clinician that careful assessment of posture and hip musculature is required when evaluating hip joint dysfunction.

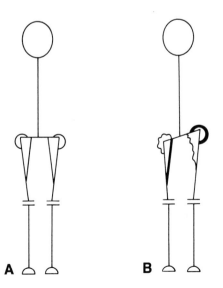

Fig. 9-3. (**A**) Symmetric stance with symmetric pull on abductor and adductor muscles. (**B**) Elevated pelvis on the right results in hip adduction on the right and abduction on the left with a stretch to the left adductors and right abductors and shortening of the left abductors and right adductors.

A   B

The discussion above presents the hip's response to static posture, but consideration should also be given to how posture, or balance, can be controlled by the hips. Three basic movement patterns have been identified in normal subjects to maintain balanced standing posture under various perturbations: ankle, hip, and stepping strategies.[13,14] In the ankle strategy the subject uses distal lower extremity musculature to move the body over the feet with little motion from the knee or hip joints. The hip strategy is employed when the ankle forces cannot adequately control the superincumbent body. When distal leg motion or ankle motion is insufficient to control the body, the subject tends to flex or extend the hips to maintain the position of the center of mass over the base of support. This strategy is used by normal subjects who sustain large perturbations to balance or when the subjects must stand on such a small support that ankle strategies are not feasible. For example, a gymnast standing on a balance beam or a diver balancing backward on the end of a diving board must resort to hip motions to maintain balance. Patients with ankle weakness also may have to utilize hip strategies for balance more frequently in the absence of dorsiflexion and plantarflexion strength to control the body above.

It was noted earlier that hip flexor strength is required to maintain quiet erect posture. However, utilization of the hip strategy to maintain balance during perturbations requires trunk and thigh musculature.[13] Rectus femoris and biceps femoris as well as erector spinae and abdominal muscles are recruited in a proximal to distal pattern to control the pelvis and hip joint. Thus, hip strength and control may influence a patient's ability to maintain balance under stressful circumstances or in the presence of distal weakness. The physical therapist must investigate the strength and integrity of the hip in the patient with balance disturbances. Conversely, the patient's ability to maintain upright balance must also be considered in the presence of hip pathology.

ROLE OF THE HIP IN LOCOMOTION

Analysis of gait includes the investigation of both kinematic parameters (displacement, velocity, and acceleration) and kinetic, or force, characteristics. The kinematic behavior of the hip is discussed first, followed by a discussion of the kinetics as applied to the hip joint.

Kinematics

The angular displacement of the hip joint during the gait cycle has been measured by many investigators using various techniques of data collection.[15-20] Murray[15] utilized stroboscopic photography to assess sagittal plane motion. Johnston and Smidt,[16] Smidt,[17] and Gore et al.[18] used electrogoniometers to determine the three-dimensional movement of the hip. Inman et al.[19] used high-speed cinematography to measure the three-dimensional motion of the hip, and Winter[20] used television to measure sagittal plane motion of the hip. Comparison of absolute measures of excursion is difficult because the researchers used different frames of reference with which to describe the movement. Murray assessed femoral movement with respect to a horizontal reference frame. Johnston, Inman, Gore, and Winter utilized body-fixed reference frames and thus assessed femoral movement with respect to the pelvis or trunk, which therefore more closely reflects true hip motion than Murray's reference frame (Fig. 9-4). However, Johnston used the standing posture of each subject as the zero or neutral position, which may or may not have been an accurate assumption. As discussed earlier, the position of the hip in quiet standing depends on both pelvic and femoral alignment. Therefore, if the subject stood in an anterior pelvic tilt, the hip is most likely in some flexion. Yet Johnston's method apparently ignored such a possibility. Despite these basic differences in approach to measurement, there is generally widespread acceptance of the overall pattern of hip joint movement in the sagittal plane during ambulation at free, or natural, speed. For purposes of consistency, the gait cycle will be considered the period of time from initial contact of one limb to the next initial contact of that same limb. At initial contact, the hip joint is flexed between 20° and 30°. It remains close to this maximally flexed position during the next 10 percent of the gait cycle while the knee is flexing and then begins to extend and continues to extend until contralateral heel strike, which occurs at 50 percent of the gait cycle. Maximum extension has been reported to be 10° to 15° of hyperextension. Following maximum hip extension, the hip resumes flexing through the end of the stance phase and most of the swing phase.[15] The hip reaches maximum hip flexion of approximately 30° shortly before initial contact or at about 85 percent of the gait cycle.

The role of pelvic motion is critical to the position of the hip during locomo-

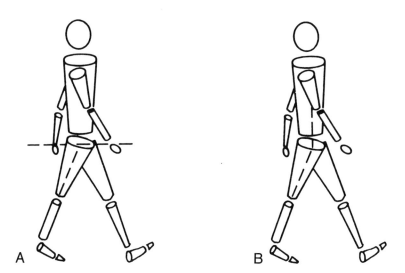

Fig. 9-4. (**A**) Reference frame with respect to the horizontal. (**B**) Reference frame with respect to the trunk.

tion. As discussed earlier, the pelvis can move over the fixed femur during quiet standing and thus affect the position of the hip joint. However, during gait the pelvis and femur can move as a single unit, so that pelvic alignment can effect femoral positioning. When the pelvis is free to move on the fixed femur, an anterior pelvic tilt results in hip joint flexion. However, when the femur and pelvis move as a unit, an anterior pelvic tilt will result in a backward inclination of the femur, which when viewed from a room-fixed reference frame will appear to be hip hyperextension (Fig. 9-5). Murray[15] noted that the pelvis reaches a maximum anterior tilt at the time of maximum hip extension, which suggests that the backward inclination of the femur at maximum hip extension is the result of true hip hyperextension, an anterior pelvic tilt, or a combination of hyperextension and pelvic tilt. The contribution of pelvic movement to femoral position in gait is magnified in the subject with a painful hip. Murray[15] reported that a patient with a painful hip demonstrated an increase in the anterior tilt of the pelvis and a marked decrease in hip extension or backward inclination of the femur in late stance. Although Murray[15] did not report the passive range of motion, Stauffer et al.[21] reported that the mean flexion contracture in 25 preoperative patients awaiting total hip replacements was 23° (the range was 0° to 80°). Therefore, it is possible that the hip extension reported in the patient with unilateral hip disease may have been the result of pelvic rotation rather than real hip hyperextension. Just as an anterior pelvic tilt can compensate for limited hip extension, a posterior pelvic tilt can be used to help advance the limb in the absence of hip flexion range of motion or strength.[22] This realization should help solidify in the minds of clinicians the interrelationship between hip and lumbar spine motion. Limited hip motion can be compensated for by increased pelvic motion.[22] However, the price for this compensation is excessive lumbar spine motion during locomotion, which could contribute to low back pain.

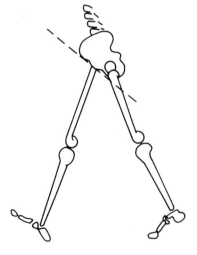

Fig. 9-5. Anterior pelvic tilt (line through ASIS and pubic symphysis) can result in a posterior projection of the femur.

Murray,[15] Crowninshield et al.,[23] and Inman et al.[19] reported an increased joint excursion in the sagittal plane with increased walking speed corresponding with increased stride length. However, both Murray and Inman noted a greater increase in hip flexion during terminal swing with little or no increase in hip extension in stance. These results suggest that the hip functions close to its end range extension during gait and that increased stride length can be accomplished only through increased hip flexion at terminal swing. Winter[20] reported very little change in joint excursion with walking speed. However, what change was reported was greater at maximum flexion than at maximum extension and suggested an increase in excursion with increased speed. While these data at first appear contradictory, I believe they reflect a difference in the magnitude of velocity effects, which may be the result of differences in the walking speeds studied. However, these variations demonstrate the need for further research to clarify velocity effects on hip joint kinematics.

There are fewer data available to describe the motion of the hip in the frontal and transverse planes during locomotion. To understand hip joint positions during gait, it must be noted again that hip joint position is the summation of pelvic and femoral alignments. The pattern or direction of movement appears consistent across subjects. However, the absolute position of the joint is quite variable.[19] This is the result of the difficulties in determining a consistent neutral position but also appears to reflect individual variability. In the frontal plane, the hip appears slightly abducted or at neutral at initial contact but moves rapidly into adduction during loading. Adduction is the result of the drop of the pelvis on the opposite, or unsupported, side but is magnified by the lateral glide of the trunk toward the supporting side. Adduction appears to reach a maximum at approximately 20 percent of the gait cycle just after single-limb stance has begun. During midstance the pelvis returns to a horizontal position, which decreases hip adduction. As the trunk shifts to the opposite side in preparation for the loading of the contralateral limb, adduction is further reduced. The hip actually moves into a position of abduction during early swing as the result of the rapid drop of the now unsupported pelvis on the ipsilateral side. As the pelvis is reoriented in midswing, the hip returns to a position of slight abduction or even neutral for initial contact again. Johnson and Smidt[16] reported a mean of 7° of abduction and 5° of adduction in 33 subjects.

Transverse plane movement of the hip joint is also small and is the summation of femoral and pelvic rotations. There appears to be considerable variability in the actual magnitudes, but the directions of the motions seem quite consistent.[19] At heel strike the hip is in slight external rotation or in neutral but moves rapidly into internal rotation during contact response. The hip remains in internal rotation through most of stance but begins to externally rotate during the last one-half or one-third of stance. The hip remains in external rotation throughout most of stance but begins to internally rotate in the latter half of swing. Johnston and Smidt[16] reported maximum excursions of 5° for both internal and external rotations.

In both transverse and frontal plane motions, excursions are very small, data are scanty, and the precision of the measurement instruments is suspect.

Therefore, the clinician should be most concerned about the direction of the hip movement. The magnitude of the movements may vary.

The kinematic data reported here were gathered from 30 men studied by Murray,[15] 33 by Johnston and Smidt,[16] an unspecified number of subjects by Inman et al.,[19] and 17 to 20 subjects by Winter.[20] Unlike the other investigators, Inman did not report descriptive data across a population. Instead he reported individual subject data. There are still very few data collected from women or from older subjects. Crowninshield et al.[23] did compare 15 older subjects (seven females and eight males) with 11 younger subjects (four females and seven males) and reported a decrease in stride length and velocity and an increase in cadence with age. Similar changes have been reported by others as well.[24,25] Some have reported a decrease in joint excursions with decreased walking velocity[20,23,26] even in young subjects. Therefore, the decreased hip motion with age reported by Crowninshield et al.[23] may reflect the decreased walking velocity characteristic of the aged subject rather than a requisite decrease in joint excursion with aging.

Hip motion during locomotion in subjects with hip pathology has been monitored by several researchers.[21,22,27–29] In general, these investigators found that walking velocity and cadence were decreased in subjects with hip pathology when compared with normal subjects. They also reported decreased joint excursion in all three planes during walking by patients with hip disease.[21,27,28] However, since decreased velocity appears to result in decreased joint excursions even in normal subjects, these data must be interpreted carefully. Total hip joint replacements have been shown to result in increased walking velocity, cadence, and joint excursion when compared with the preoperative status.[21,27] However, these subjects still did not return to normal gait performances.

At this point, the clinician must ask what these data mean in practice. First, hip pathology can be expected to le. to gait abnormalities. Second, among the gait deviations to be expected is decreased velocity. With decreased velocity, changes in joint excursions may be anticipated and have been reported. However, improvements in joint excursions are unlikely without an increase in walking velocity. Yet, as demonstrated in the following section on joint kinetics, increased walking velocity may increase the load on the hip joint and therefore may increase pain. Thus, the patient may be in a vicious cycle of decreased velocity and decreased joint excursions that can only be interrupted by decreasing the stress on the joint. It behooves the clinician to consider this interrelationship when intervening in gait and when considering assistive devices.

Joint Kinetics

This segment discussed the forces applied to the hip joint during ambulation and the controlling mechanisms of the hip joint that may influence the efficiency of gait. Forces at the hip joint during normal locomotion are generally derived from mathematical analysis of the movement since direct measurement of joint reaction forces in normal individuals is not available. Paul[30] used Newtonian mechanics to calculate the reaction force on the femoral head in normal men and women during locomotion. He found that the force peaked twice in stance in both men and women, once following initial contact and again before toe off. The mean of the first peak was approximately four times body weight in men and approximately two and one-half times body weight in women. The second peak was substantially larger, approximately seven times body weight in men and four times body weight in women. Paul[30] reported that these peaks corresponded to bursts of activity of the abductor muscles stabilizing the pelvis.

In any mechanical analysis of joint forces, a solution requires that the number of unknown quantities such as joint reaction forces and moments and muscle forces and moments equal the number of equations available to describe the movement. In a three-dimensional system there are three joint reaction forces along the three axes and three moments about the three axes and there are six equations of motion describing the system. Seireg and Arvikar[31] listed 16 muscles that cross the hip joint and could potentially apply a force to the hip. Thus, there are a total of 22 unknowns in a system with six equations of motion. There are more unknowns than equations, which results in an infinite number of possible solutions. Such a system is said to be indeterminant. To avoid this situation, Paul[30] and others have made simplifying assumptions to reduce the number of unknowns by considering only large muscle groups and ignoring simultaneous activity of two or more muscles. Such assumptions, which were necessary for solving the problem, have not accurately represented the muscle activity during locomotion. Therefore, the data resulting from such analysis can be regarded as estimates at best. This procedure has been utilized to assess the kinetic parameters of other activities of daily living. Fleckenstein et al.[32] used a similar approach to calculate hip joint moments while rising from sitting to standing and reported significantly larger hip joint extension moments when rising with the knees flexed to 75° than when rising with the knees flexed to 105°. Thus, this approach helps provide a perspective on the effects of activities of daily living on joint forces and gives some indication of the implications of movement dysfunction.

To avoid making such apparently questionable assumptions, some have utilized optimization techniques to choose the "best" solution from the infinite number of possibilities.[31,33] The "best" solution is chosen based on optimization criteria such as minimizing the sum of the muscle forces and joint moments. These investigators reported values of hip joint reaction forces similar to those reported by Paul.[30]

While joint forces cannot be measured in vivo in normal subjects, instrumented implants have enabled investigators to measure hip joint forces in postoperative patients. Rydell[34] implanted an instrumented femoral head replacement in two patients. Measured forces were less than those calculated values reported for normal subjects but remained substantial. Forces of almost three times body weight were reported in fast walking. Rydell[34] also recorded forces on the femoral head during hip flexion while supine and during extension while prone that were larger than loads during very slow walking. Nordin and Frankel[35] reported hip joint forces derived from an instrumented nail plate used after a hip fracture osteotomy. They suggested that bed mobility activities such as raising the buttocks onto a bedpan resulted in loads similar to those developed in walking. Even foot and ankle exercises produced increased femoral head forces.

These data demonstrate that the hip joint sustains very large loads repeatedly during activities of daily living. If repeated loading can influence the degenerative process in diseased joints, the physical therapist must be mindful of the loads applied to the joint during exercise and activities of daily living. In addition, joint loading in a damaged joint appears to increase pain. Therefore therapists must seek ways to minimize joint loading to minimize the patient's pain.

Joint reaction forces are equal and opposite to the other forces applied to the body segment such as muscle forces and ground reaction forces. To understand the magnitude of the joint reaction forces, it is necessary to understand the role of the muscles in stabilizing and propelling the hip during locomotion. Inman et al.[19] noted that the majority of muscle activity in gait occurs at the transitions between stance and swing and between swing and stance. The lower extremity is accelerating or decelerating rapidly at these times and body weight is being shifted either onto or off the limb.

The role of the abductors (gluteus medius and minimus) is to stabilize the pelvis during stance.[19,20,36] In addition, they may contribute to advancement of the pelvis over the stance limb in the transverse plane. They are active generally from just before initial contact to initial contact on the opposite side. Since the pelvis drops after initial contact, the abductors contract in a lengthened condition to control and then reverse the descent of the pelvis.

The gluteus maximus is active at initial contact into early stance as the hip moves from its maximally flexed position and begins to extend.[19,20,36] Thus the gluteus maximus appears to control hip and pelvic flexion and may contribute to hip extension as the trunk moves over the femur. The hamstrings are also active at initial contact into early stance, assisting in hip extension. The activity of the gluteus maximus and the hamstrings actually begins in late swing, apparently to decelerate the flexion of the hip and extension of the knee. Winter[20] also reported a short burst of activity in these muscles in early swing to begin the deceleration. It must be recognized that the hip continues to extend through midstance despite the lack of any continued activity in the gluteus maximus and hamstrings. It appears that the gluteus maximus and hamstrings provide a braking, or deceleration, action and perhaps some initial thrust into extension but the motion is continued by some other force or by forward momentum.

Activity of the iliacus[19] is demonstrated at late stance and early swing as the hip reverses its motion from extension into flexion. Again hip flexion continues through most of swing long after iliacus activity has ceased. Quadriceps[19,20,36] activity has also been demonstrated in some subjects at toe off that may reflect rectus femoris activity to assist the iliacus in decelerating and then accelerating the femur. Of course, the quadriceps are also active in early stance to control knee flexion. The tensor fasciae latae[19] is active at terminal stance and terminal swing. Its activity at terminal stance has been attributed to its role as a hip flexor with the iliacus. Its activity at terminal swing may be to balance the effects of gluteus maximus activity on the iliotibial band and to increase frontal plane stability with the gluteus medius.

Adductor activity during gait seems more variable. However, recording adductor activity during locomotion is technically more difficult than in other muscles because the advancing limb tends to rub the electrodes against each other. However, activity has been found in these muscles at both the beginning and end of swing.[19,20,36] Eberhart et al.[36] and Winter[20] also noted activity of the adductors during early stance. Activity during swing suggests that the adductors assist in both limb acceleration and deceleration as well as control of the swing limb in the frontal plane. Stance-phase activity supports the adductors' responsibility in stabilizing the pelvis with the hip abductors and extensors.

The critical element in understanding the role of the hip musculature during gait is to recognize the brevity of each muscle's activity. These data emphasize the efficiency of locomotion in normal subjects in which very brief activation of a muscle can slow, reverse, or propel the limb but is not required then to maintain that motion. The hip plays an important part in controlling locomotion and contributing to its efficiency. The following presents the theories of the controlling mechanisms in gait and the hip's role in energy conservation.

The realization that very little muscle activity is present during the swing phase of gait has led investigators to compare the movement of the lower extremity with that of a compound or jointed pendulum.[37,38] In this model, the limb has a set of initial conditions, that is, initial position and velocity, and then is allowed to swing acted on only by gravity. These investigators found that such a model presented a displacement and force history of the lower extremity consistent with the swing limb of normal subjects. Mena et al.[39] elaborated on this model and investigated the effect of certain clinically measurable parameters of gait on the predicted movement of the limb. They found that the pattern of movement of the swing limb was most dependent on the angular velocity of the thigh. In other words, normal hip joint movement resulted in normal predicted movements of the leg and foot. Conversely, abnormal movements of the hip predicted significantly abnormal patterns of movement of the leg and foot. Although these data are artificially generated utilizing a mathematical model of the lower extremity, data reported by Godges et al.[40] lend indirect clinical support for such a model. They compared two methods of stretching to increase hip range of motion and then evaluated the effect of increased hip flexibility on oxygen consumption in brisk walking and in running at two different speeds. A significant decrease in oxygen consumption was noted at all three speeds following stretching. There are a variety of possible explanations to explain these results. However, one possible explanation is that increased range resulted in a more normal thigh trajectory in swing, thus improving the patterns of movement of the leg and foot, consequently reducing energy expenditure.

Investigating the mechanical energy exchange within and between limb segments can also help in understanding the importance of the hip and thigh in regulating the pattern and efficiency of gait. There are two forms of mechanical energy. Kinetic energy is a function of the segment's velocity (linear or rotational), and potential energy is a function of the height of the segment's center of gravity from the ground.[19] The principle of conversation of energy states that a change in the total energy of a segment, that is, the sum of kinetic and potential energy, requires that work be done on the segment. Thus, a transfer of energy from one form to another implies efficiency of movement since the total energy remains the same. Winter et al.[41] investigated the energy transfer within the torso, thigh, and shank. They demonstrated that the torso exchanges about one-half of its energy, the thigh exchanges approximately one-third of its energy, and the shank exhibited almost no exchange. Later research investigated the possibility of an energy exchange between segments.[42] This concept is loosely analogous to children playing crack-the-whip, in which energy is transferred from the leader down the line of children. Because the joint reaction force has an equal and opposite value for adjacent articulating surfaces, it follows that an input of energy at one segment is accompanied by an outflow of energy at the adjacent segment. Winter and Robertson[43] reported that energy is transmitted to and from the hip particularly at the beginning and end of the swing phase of gait, facilitating the acceleration and deceleration of the leg and foot.

Analysis of power, which is the product of force and velocity (torque and angular velocity in rotational movements), has also been useful in demonstrating the role muscles play in generating and absorbing energy. Winter[20] stated that positive power represented a concentric muscle contraction and negative power indicated an eccentric contraction. This analysis again yields data that demonstrate the role of the hip flexors and extensors in driving and controlling the entire lower extremity. The role of two-joint muscles in the lower extremity in allowing such energy flow between segments was also addressed by Wells.[44] Using an analysis similar to that reported by Winter et al.[41] Wells[44] reported that the two-joint muscles of the lower extremity including the hamstrings and quadriceps could account for a mean savings in work of 11.6 percent with a range of 7 to 29 percent over a similar movement pattern produced by one-joint muscles.

The data presented above were mathematically generated to analyze the mechanisms dictating the efficiency of gait. What meaning does this theoretical information have for the clinician? These studies are presented here to provide a perspective regarding the role of the hip in locomotion. Much earlier in this chapter, studies were presented documenting the gait dysfunctions that occur in the presence of hip pathology. However, most clinicians already acknowledge that hip pain results in an antalgic gait. The gait studies serve primarily to verify our clinical observations. However, the models of locomotion presented here may help us to realize that the hip is not just an isolated joint moving through its rather simple pattern of movement during gait. Rather it appears to be at least part of the driving force for the whole lower extremity. In addition, it is controlled by two-joint muscles that in turn help to conserve energy throughout the lower extremity. Thus, hip pathology will result in more than just abnormal behavior of the hip joint in gait. It can alter the kinematic and kinetic parameters of the lower extremities and the whole body. Thus, the data presented by Brown et al.[29] should not surprise us. Brown et al.[29] reported a significant increase in oxygen consumption during ambulation in subjects with unilateral and bilateral hip disease when compared with normal subjects. After total hip joint replacement, these subjects exhibited improved but still abnormal oxygen consumption. In view of the hip's importance in influencing other joint motions, altered gait velocity and joint excursions can have only negative and substantial effects on energy expenditure. Thus, the clinician must remain mindful of the extent of movement dysfunction that is likely with hip joint pathology.

SUMMARY

The hip joint has a well-characterized pattern of movement during locomotion controlled by an equally repeatable pattern of muscle activity. In addition, there is strong evidence that the hip also affects the performance of other joints during locomotion. Thus, the physical therapist must examine the hip in isolation and within the context of the whole body in motion to evaluate the extent of the dysfunction and consequently to effect a positive change.

REFERENCES

1. Turner M: Posture and pain. Phys Ther 37:294, 1957
2. Steindler A: Kinesiology of the Human Body under Normal and Pathological Conditions. Charles C Thomas, Springfield, IL, 1955
3. Kendall FP, McCreary EK: Muscles, Testing and Function. 3rd Ed. Williams & Wilkins, Baltimore, 1983
4. Harty M: The anatomy of the hip joint. p. 45. In Tronzo RG (ed): Surgery of the Hip Joint. Vol. 1. Springer-Verlag, New York, 1984
5. Soderberg GL: Kinesiology, Application to Pathological Motion. Williams & Wilkins, Baltimore, 1986
6. Day JW, Smidt GL, Lehmann T: Effect of pelvic tilt on standing posture. Phys Ther 64:510, 1984
7. Gajdosik R, Simpson R, Smith R, DonTigny R: Pelvic tilt, intratester reliability of measuring the standing position and range of motion. Phys Ther 65:169, 1985
8. Basmajian JV: Muscles Alive, Their Functions Revealed by Electromyography. 2nd Ed. Williams & Wilkins, Baltimore, 1967
9. Edberg E: Bracing for patients with traumatic paraplegia. p. 50. In Perry J, Hislop HJ (eds): Principles of Lower-Extremity Bracing. American Physical Therapy Association, Washington, DC, 1967
10. Neumann DA, Soderberg GL, Cook TM: Comparison of maximal isometric hip abductor muscles torques between hip sides. Phys Ther 68:596, 1988
11. Bourbon D: Hand dominance and its effects on postural asymmetries and selected muscle weakness. Master of Science thesis. Beaver College, Glenside, PA, 1987
12. Gossman MR, Sahrman SA, Rose SJ: Review of length-associated changes in muscle. Phys Ther 62:1799, 1982
13. Horak FB, Sashner LM: Central programming of postural movements: Adaptation to altered support-surface configurations. Neurophysiol 55:1369, 1986
14. Horak FB: Clinical measurement of postural control in adults. Phys Ther 67:1881, 1987

15. Murray MP: Gait as a total pattern of movement, including a bibliography on gait. Am J Phys Med 48:290, 1967
16. Johnston RC, Smidt GL: Measurement of hip joint motion during walking: Evaluation of an electrogoniometric method. J Bone Joint Surg 51A:1083, 1969
17. Smidt GL: Hip motion and related factors in walking. Phys Ther 51:9, 1971
18. Gore TA, Flynn M, Stevens J: Measurement and analysis of hip joint movements. Institute of Mechanical Engineers 8:21, 1978
19. Inman VT, Ralston HJ, Todd F: Human Walking. Williams & Wilkins, Baltimore, 1981
20. Winter DA: The Biomechanics and Motor Control of Human Gait. University of Waterloo Press, Waterloo, Ontario, Canada, 1987
21. Stauffer RN, Smidt GL, Wadsworth JB: Clinical and biomechanical analysis of gait following Charnley total hip replacement. Clin Orthop 99:70, 1974
22. Gore DR, Murray MP, Sepic SB, Gardner GM: Walking patterns of men with unilateral surgical hip fusion. J Bone Joint Surg 57:759, 1975
23. Crowninshield RD, Brand RA, Johnston RC: The effects of walking velocity and age on hip kinematics and kinetics. Clin Orthop 132:140, 1978
24. Finley FR, Cody KA, Finizie RV: Locomotion patterns in elderly women. Arch Phys Med 50:140, 1969
25. Murray MP, Kory KC, Clarkson BH: Walking patterns in healthy old men. J Gerontol 24:169, 1969
26. Craik R, Herman R, Finley FR: Human solutions for locomotion: Interlimb coordination. Adv Behav Biol 18:51, 1976
27. Murray MP, Brewer BJ, Zuege RD: Kinesiologic measurements of functional performance before and after McKee-Ferrar total hip replacement. J Bone Joint Surg 54A:237, 1972
28. Wadsworth JB, Smidt GL, Johnston RC: Gait characteristics of subjects with hip disease. Phys Ther 52:829, 1972
29. Brown M, Hislop HJ, Waters RL, Porell D: Walking efficiency before and after total hip replacement. Phys Ther 60:1259, 1980
30. Paul JP: Forces transmitted by joints in the human body. Proc Inst Mech Eng 181:8, 1967
31. Seireg A, Arvikar RJ: The prediction of muscular load sharing and joint forces in the lower extremities during walking. J Biomech 8:89, 1975
32. Fleckenstein SJ, Dirby RL, MacLeod DA: Effects of limited knee-flexion range on peak hip moments of force while transferring from sitting to standing. J Biomech 21:915, 1988
33. Crowninshield RD, Johnston RC, Andrews JG, Brand RA: A biomechanical investigation of the human hip. J Biomech 11:75, 1978
34. Rydell N: Forces in the hip joint. Part II. Intravital measurement. p. 351. In Kenedi RM (ed): Biomechanics and Related Bio-Engineering Topics. Pergamon Press, Oxford, 1965
35. Nordin M, Frankel VH: Biomechanics of the hip. p. 149. In Frankel VH, Nordin M (eds): Basic Biomechanics of the Skeletal System. Lea & Febiger, Philadelphia, 1980
36. Eberhart HD, Inman VT, Saunders JB, et al: Fundamental studies of human locomotion and other information relating to design of artificial limbs. A Report to the National Research Council, Committee on Artificial Limbs. University of California, Berkley, 1947
37. Mochon S, McMahon TA: Ballistic walking. J Biomech 13:49, 1980.
38. McMahon TA: Muscles, Reflexes, and Locomotion. Princeton University Press, Princeton, 1984

39. Mena D, Mansour JM, Simon SR: Analysis and synthesis of human swing leg motion during gait and its clinical applications. J Biomech 14:823, 1981
40. Godges JJ, MacRae H, Longdon C, et al: The effects of two stretching procedures on hip range of motion and gait economy. J Orthop Sports Phys Ther 10:350, 1989
41. Winter DA, Quanbury AO, Reimer GD: Analysis of instantaneous energy of normal gait. J Biomech 9:253, 1976
42. Robertson DGE, Winter DA: Mechanical energy generation, absorption, and transfer amongst segments druing walking. J Biomech 13:845, 1980
43. Winter DA, Robertson DGE: Joint torque and energy patterns in normal gait. Biol Cybern 29:137, 1978
44. Wells RP: Mechanical energy costs of human movement: An approach to evaluating the transfer possibilities of two-joint muscles. J Biomech 21:955, 1988

10 | Hip Problems in Children and Adolescents

Deborah King-Echternach

"When I look upon a child I am filled with admiration, not so much for what that child is today as for what it may become."[1] This quote by Louis Pasteur reminds us as pediatric physical therapists that we have a unique opportunity to impose change on a developing musculoskeletal system. It must be remembered that children are not just small adults but are different owing to the immaturity of their bodily systems.

Bony configuration of the hip in the newborn is notably different from that in the adult. Normally, at birth, the femoral neck-shaft angle, or angle of inclination, is approximately 150°.[2,3] With normal weightbearing and growth, this angle usually decreases to 130° by early adulthood.[2,4] The condition of an increased neck-shaft angle is referred to as coxa valga, while a decreased angle is known as coxa vara. Infants display a greater degree of anteversion, in which the femoral neck is angled anteriorly to the long axis of the femoral shaft. This angle decreases to 15° in the adult.[5]

Mechanical forces on the musculoskeletal system can affect both size and shape of the body parts.[3,6] Poor positioning and muscle imbalance can modify the structure of bone and cause deformation. Careful management of these deforming forces is critical, especially during growth periods, to retard or reverse their ill effects.

Normal variations of the skeletal components making up the hip that occur in children may spontaneously correct with age.[1,7] Two such conditions are external and internal femoral torsion. These rotational variations may result from repeated twisting forces along the epiphyseal plates. Habitual positioning in the prone position with externally rotated hips may exacerbate external femoral torsion, while the reversed tailor or W position may promote excessive internal femoral torsion. Scoles[7] states that in normal children, spontaneous correction occurs without therapeutic intervention. Salter,[1] however, believes that intervention including tailor positioning and possibly a night brace may aid in the correction of internal femoral torsion.

Hip problems in children and adolescents may be classified as congenital, developmental, disease processes, and traumatic.

CONGENITAL HIP PROBLEMS

Congenital hip abnormalities are present at birth and are characterized by abnormal skeletal growth and development or joint instability. Congenital hip disease may include dysplasia, subluxation, and dislocation. Dysplasia describes an abnormal relationship of the acetabulum and femoral head from bony remodeling. A steep acetabular roof and small femoral head are signs of dysplasia.[7]

Congenital Hip Dislocation

The incidence of congenital hip subluxation and dislocation (CHD) is 1.5:1,000 and affects girls eight times more frequently than boys.[1] CHD is considered *teratologic* when the condition develops in utero and *typical* when it appears postnatally. Mechanical, physiologic, and environmental factors may contribute to CHD.

Mechanical factors include restricted intrauterine space and breech presentation. Physiologic factors are related to laxity of the pelvic joint and hip capsule in the newborn from maternal estrogens. Postnatal environmental factors such as maintained hip extension in the newborn or sudden passive extension immediately after birth may contribute to CHD.[1,6-8]

Early diagnosis and treatment of typical CHD is critical, since a dislocated hip may be easily reduced before secondary changes occur. These secondary changes include acetabular dysplasia, femoral anteversion, hypertrophy of the capsule, and muscle contracture.[1,8]

Diagnosis may be confirmed by radiographs (Fig. 10-1) and a positive Ortolani and Barlow test (see Ch. 2). Passive abduction is usually limited, and an increase in external rotation is noted. There may also be an increase in the number of skin folds of the medial thigh. In the older child, shortening of the limb, a telescoping femur, and a positive Trendelenburg test are usually found.

When CHD is diagnosed in the neonate, treatment usually consists of splinting in abduction such as the Pavlik harness or Frejka pillow following reduction (Fig. 10-1C & D). The duration of splinting depends on how soon after the problem was discovered splinting was first applied.[8]

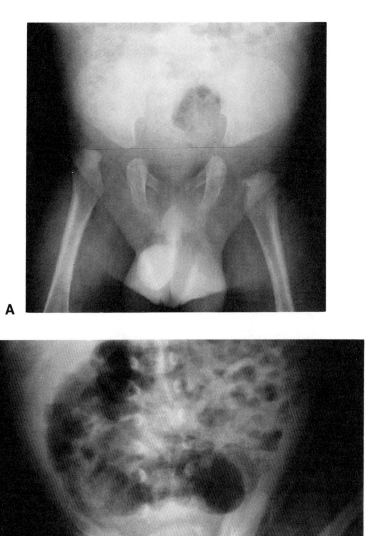

Fig. 10-1. (**A**) Radiograph of 2-month-old child with bilateral CHD before treatment. (**B**) Radiograph of 4-week-old child with CHD in Frejka pillow. (*Figure continues.*)

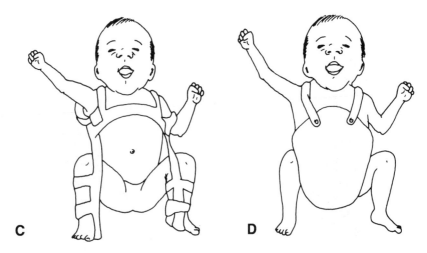

Fig. 10-1 (*Continued*).   (**C**) Pavlik harness for CHD. (**D**) Frejka pillow for CHD.

In an older child, when the hip cannot be reduced owing to contracture and bony changes, traction and cast reduction are indicated. Open reduction and an adductor tenotomy may be needed if the diagnosis is made after a child is of walking age.[1]

If muscle imbalance or gait deviations are present in a child who has undergone surgery for CHD, physical therapy is indicated. Upper extremity and trunk strengthening may begin while the child is in a cast. After cast removal, mobilization and strengthening of the hips and knees may be initiated along with progressive weightbearing ambulation. A warm pool is an excellent medium to begin the physical therapy program.

Congenital Coxa Vara

Coxa vara is a bony defect in the femoral neck causing a decrease in the angle of inclination and shortening of the limb. It is frequently bilateral, producing a duck waddle gait. If unilateral, a positive Trendelenburg test may be found on the affected side along with limited abduction and internal rotation. Treatment of coxa vara may include protection against excessive weight-bearing, strengthening of the abductors, and measures to equalize leg length. If deformity is severe, an abduction subtrochanteric osteotomy may be indicated.[1,4]

DEVELOPMENTAL HIP PROBLEMS

Developmental hip disorders are gradually acquired owing to a condition present at or shortly after birth that affects growth and development. This may include cerebral palsy, spina bifida, arthrogryposis and genetic disorders.

Cerebral Palsy

Cerebral palsy (CP) is a nonprogressive disorder of the central nervous system that impairs normal motor development. It affects one to five children per thousand.[9] Several types and distributions may be found. Most types of CP have a spastic component, characterized by cocontraction of agonist and antagonist muscle groups. Although bone and joint structure is normal at birth, joint contractures and dislocations may develop because of imbalance and overactivity of these spastic muscles. Deformities of the hip may interfere with sitting and ambulation and predispose the hip to fractures and disabling pain.[10,11] Early intervention to detect the etiology of hip dysfunction and provide preventative and corrective measures is essential.

Hip instability in CP is an acquired condition reflecting persistence of fetal hip structure (neck valgus and increased femoral anteversion) resulting from delayed weightbearing.[10] Strong hip flexors and adductors frequently overpower the abductors and extensors leading to dislocation (Fig. 10-2A). Dislocation is more common in the nonambulatory and quadriplegic CP child and may begin as early as 3 years of age.[11]

The windblown hip syndrome consists of three major factors: dislocation of the hip followed by pelvic obliquity and finally scoliosis.[12] The pelvis is usually tilted upward on the side of the dislocation, with a convex scoliosis away from that side (Fig. 10-2B). As this deformity progresses, seating and treatment become more difficult.

Evaluation of the hip in CP should include assessment of muscle tone, reflexes, and range of motion (ROM) of pelvis, hip, and knee; tests for femoral anteversion; observation of patterns of movement during functional activities; and gait analysis.

Management of hip problems should include attempts at tone reduction, ROM, achievement of good postural alignment in a variety of positions, and facilitation of normal movement patterns. When these conservative measures fail to prevent a developing deformity, surgical intervention is often indicated.

Surgical procedures may include soft tissue releases (adductors, iliopsoas, hamstring muscles), varus rotation osteotomy, and obturator neurectomy. In an older child with a shallow dysplastic acetabulum, a Chiari or other pelvic osteotomy may be indicated. In the adolescent or young adult over 18 years of age with a chronic dislocation, response to surgical intervention is often poor.[9] For the painful dislocated hip in the young adult, a hip arthodesis or total hip replacement may be considered as a salvage procedure.[10]

Myelomeningocele

Another group at risk for development of a hip problem is the child with myelomeningocele. As the result of a neural tube defect, the child loses neuromotor control below the level of the lesion. Muscle imbalance, postural effects of gravity, and weightbearing may lead to limb deformity. A child with func-

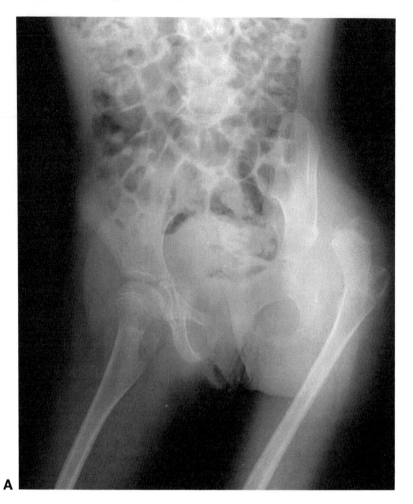

A

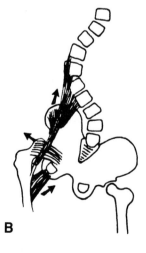

B

Fig. 10-2. (**A**) Radiograph of fixed adduction and flexion with increasing pelvic obliquity and hip dislocation in CP child, age 9 years. (**B**) The role of the iliopsoas in the production of the wind-blown hip syndrome. (Fig. B from Letts et al.,[12] with permission.)

tional hip flexors and adductors accompanied by paralysis of the hip extensors and abductors is at risk for hip instability and dislocation.[13]

Management of hip instability and deformity associated with myelomeningocele varies depending on the level of the lesion.[13–15] The child with a lesion above the 12th thoracic level is usually nonambulatory, experiences no pain with hip dislocation, and therefore is not a candidate for corrective hip surgery.[14] Conservative measures may include ROM and positioning techniques to prevent deformity. Soft tissue releases may be indicated to correct fixed contracture.

Open reduction to contain the femoral head is contraindicated in the child with an upper lumbar lesion and hip dislocation since this would not improve the child's function.[13] ROM, positioning techniques, orthotics to provide stability in standing, and gait training are helpful. Leg length discrepancies should be corrected by a shoe lift to provide for proper postural alignment (Fig. 10-3). With a good orthotic device, a child with a dislocated hip may continue standing and gait activities.

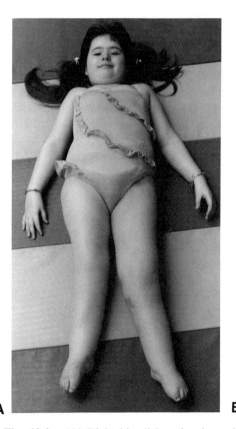 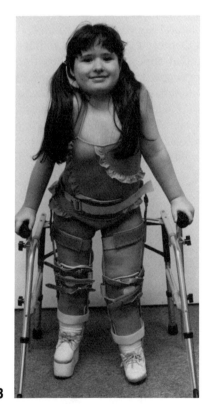

A   **B**

Fig. 10-3. (**A**) Right hip dislocation in a child with myelomeningocele at the upper lumbar level. (**B**) Same child with orthoses and shoe lift.

A child with a lower lumbar lesion, functioning quadriceps, and a good potential for household or community ambulation may be a candidate for major hip surgery.[13,15] Muscle imbalance may be corrected by iliopsoas transfer and adductor release. Weisl et al.[15] found that a varus-rotation osteotomy could be an alternative to the iliopsoas transfer for hip stabilization. A capsulorrhaphy and acetabuloplasty may also be required.

In a study by Sherk et al.,[14] no benefit was found in surgical intervention for hip dislocation in ambulatory myelomeningocele patients. Risks of surgery included postoperative pathologic fractures, ankylosis, infection, and decubitus ulcers. Despite fairly successful surgical intervention, the majority of patients relied on wheelchairs for mobility.[15] Social reasons such as more independence, improved mobility, and greater efficiency in activities of daily living may contribute to the decision by adolescents to give up walking.

Arthogryposis

Arthogryposis is a condition present at birth that involves fibrous ankylosis of multiple joints. The incidence of hip dislocation in this population varies from 14 to 42 percent.[16] In unilateral dislocations, an open reduction using an anterolateral approach is recommended to prevent pelvic obliquity and scoliosis. Staheli et al.,[16] however, found that ROM and function were greater using a medial approach. Advantages of the medial approach included minimal dissection with little scarring and a reduced casting period of 5 to 6 weeks. If ROM is adequate and the pelvis is level, bilateral dislocations are often left untreated.

Children with genetic disorders including Turner's, Wolf-Hirschhorn, cri du chat, Hurler, and Lesch-Nyhan syndromes are predisposed to developing hip dislocations.[17] They may also benefit from conservative and surgical intervention as previously described.

DISEASE PROCESSES

Several childhood diseases may contribute to hip joint dysfunction and may be specific to the hip (Legg-Calvé-Perthes disease) or may involve multiple joint dysfunction (juvenile rheumatoid arthritis).

Legg-Calvé-Perthes Disease

Legg-Calvé-Perthes disease, also known as coxa plana and juvenile osteochondrosis, is a disorder involving avascular necrosis of the femoral head. It is most frequent in children between the ages of 3 and 12, affecting boys four times more frequently than girls. Bilateral involvement is noted in approximately 15 percent of the cases. Legg-Calvé-Perthes disease has also been correlated with a low birth weight.[18]

The precise etiology of Legg-Calvé-Perthes disease is unknown, but most agree the process initially involves avascular necrosis of the epiphysis. Possible causes may include an abnormal vascular configuration, trauma, infection, and metabolic bone disease.

Legg-Calvé-Perthes disease is a self-limiting disorder that may involve all or part of the femoral head. According to Salter,[1] the natural history may be divided into four stages and take from 2 to 8 years to complete. The first phase involves necrosis resulting from avascularity, and symptoms are usually absent. In the second phase, resorption of dead bone and formation of new living bone occurs by revascularization. A fracture of the subchondral bone may occur, causing pain, effusion, and decreased ROM in the hip joint. In this phase, as remodeling occurs the new bone is vulnerable to all forces acting on it (Fig. 10-4A). The third phase involves continued bone formation, and modeling may continue without further bone resorption (Fig. 10-4B). Once healing is complete (phase four), the bone contour is established. Any malformation of the head remains unchanged, which may lead to degenerative joint disease in adulthood.[1,18] (Fig. 10-4C).

Clinically, symptoms may include an antalgic gait, muscle spasm, pain, and decreased ROM. Pain may be referred to the medial thigh or knee. Hip abduction and internal rotation are usually the most limited motions, and a flexion-adduction contracture may develop.

Protection of the softened femoral head from abnormal forces during revascularization is the primary treatment goal. Keeping the hip in abduction and slight internal rotation by means of a brace or cast assists with containment of the femoral head during the remodeling process. Abduction plaster casts, a stirrup crutch, and the Scottish Rite or Bobechko brace are frequently used (Fig. 10-4D–G). According to Salter,[1] weightbearing is not considered appropriate during remodeling if containment of the femoral head can be maintained. Before deformation occurs, a femoral osteotomy and innominate osteotomy may be an alternative to splinting. Observation may be all that is required in mild cases without subluxation that involve less than one-half of the femoral head.[1,4]

The physical therapist's initial involvement with these patients may be for gait training with crutches, which may be used with an abduction orthotic or cast. After healing is complete and cast or braces have been removed, physical therapy may be indicated to increase ROM of the hip, knee, and ankle. Pool therapy, bicycle, and Swiss ball activities may be helpful.

Slipped Capital Femoral Epiphysis

Slipping of the capital femoral epiphysis or adolescent coxa vara may be found in some children, more frequently in boys between 10 and 16 years of age.[2,4,18] The femoral head commonly slips in a posterior and inferior direction from the neck. This condition is noted more often at the time of puberty and is associated with a period of rapid growth before the epiphyseal plate closes. It is frequently seen in both obese and very slender children and may occur bilaterally.[2,4,18]

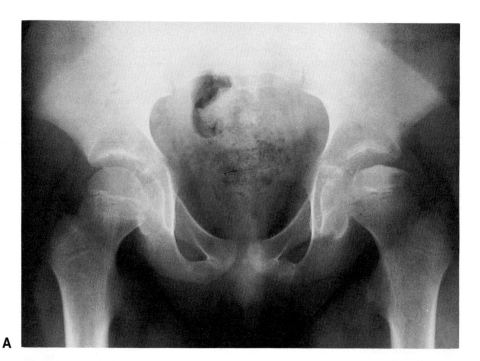

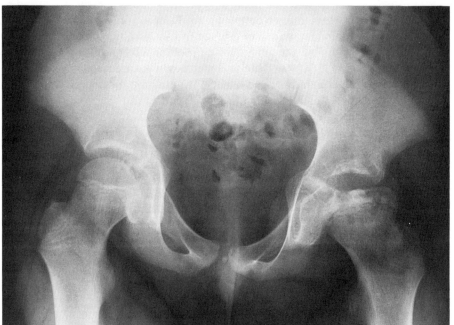

Fig. 10-4. (**A**) Radiograph of subchondral fracture during revascularization phase in child (age 9 years) with Legg-Calvé-Perthes disease. (**B**) Radiograph of same child 1 year later (age 10). (*Figure continues.*)

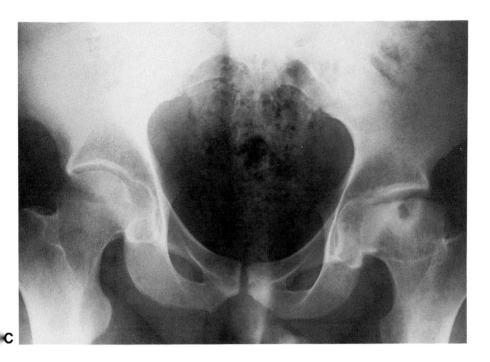

C

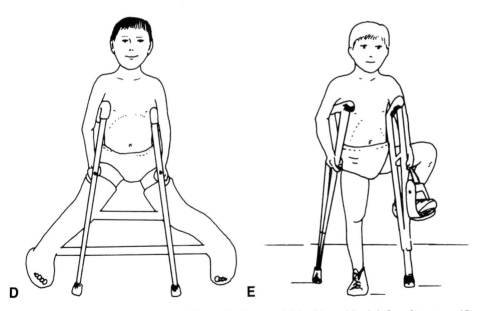

D   E

Fig. 10-4 (*Continued*).   (**C**) Radiograph of same child with residual deformity at age 19.
(**D**) Abduction plaster cast (Petrie). (**E**) Stirrup crutch treatment. (*Figure continues*.)

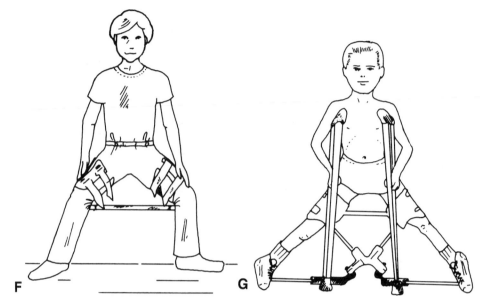

Fig. 10-4 (*Continued*). (**F**) Scottish rite abduction brace. (**G**) Abduction brace (Bobechko).

Slipped capital femoral epiphysis differs pathologically from a physeal fracture, and some studies have shown that a growth plate abnormality precedes slippage.[7] The epiphyseal plate may be displaced acutely from trauma, but chronic slippage is more common.

Clinical findings may include hip or knee pain, antalgic gait, and stiffness. Limited motion in hip internal rotation, abduction, and flexion is commonly noted. When the hip is passively flexed, the femur abducts and externally rotates.

A traumatic slipped epiphysis may occur in the newborn.[18] The neonate may avoid movement because of pain. The limb may be swollen, shortened, and externally rotated. Diagnosis can be confirmed by radiograph or bone scan.

Surgical intervention is required to prevent further slippage. The epiphyseal plate may be stabilized by thread wires or bone pegs.[18] Chondrolysis, an acute articular cartilage necrosis, may be a complication, requiring a hip fusion or total hip replacement.

Postsurgical treatment resembles methods commonly used when treating a hip fracture. Crutches to ensure non-weightbearing may be needed for several months.[4] Gait training, ROM, and strengthening activities will assist in improving function.

Juvenile Rheumatoid Arthritis

Juvenile rheumatoid arthritis (JRA), or Still's disease, is a childhood disease characterized by chronic synovial inflammation. The cause is unknown. It is more prevalent in girls and affects between 60,000 and 200,000 children in the

United States.[19] It is generally symmetric, affecting multiple joints. JRA may affect epiphyseal growth around the affected joints. The lower limbs are frequently involved, and early hip joint dysfunction is common.

Secondary osteoarthritis with sclerosis, joint space narrowing, and osteophyte formation is a common late affect of JRA. JRA of the hip may lead to coxa valga, subluxation, and compressive fractures.[20] Osteoarthritis may develop from hip joint incongruency, and a total hip replacement in adulthood may be needed.

Symptoms include morning stiffness and mild joint pain. Affected joints may be swollen, warm, and tender. Treatment goals include maintenance of joint position, strength, and function. In addition to medical management, physical therapy is indicated to provide a therapeutic program to maintain ROM, strength, and function. Positioning in the prone position will help to prevent hip flexion contracture. The child should be encouraged to remain as active and independent as possible.

Transient Synovitis

Transient synovitis is a benign and short-lived disease. Synovial membrane hypertrophy and inflammation are common findings. It is frequently found in boys 3 to 10 years of age and most always a unilateral condition.[4,18] The etiology is unknown but may be related to infection or mild trauma.[4]

Symptoms include hip pain, joint tenderness, antalgic gait, and limited hip ROM associated with muscle spasm. The child may be more comfortable in the supine position with the hip flexed and externally rotated since this position allows for maximum synovial fluid capacity in the joint. Radiographs may show joint effusion but are otherwise negative.

Treatment includes bed rest with heat and massage to the affected area until full painless ROM has returned. Recovery usually takes place within 1 week. Salter[1] recommends partial weightbearing with crutches for an additional few weeks to prevent recurrence. Because transient synovitis may contribute to the development of Legg-Calvé-Perthes disease, semiannual radiographs are recommended for a few years after the synovitis.

Septic Hip

Septic hip is an infection of the joint and synovium that may lead to articular cartilage and vascular damage if untreated. Sepsis may be caused by bacteremia from a distant infection or as a complication of a transfusion into the umbilical artery (in neonates).[18]

Symptoms include fever, swelling of the proximal thigh, and pain with movement. The limb is frequently held in flexion, abduction, and external rotation. Microorganisms such as *Staphylococcus* may be detected in aspirated joint fluid.

Treatment includes aspiration of the joint fluid followed by an arthrotomy to debride and drain the hip joint. Antibiotics are utilized but alone cannot cure septic arthritis.[18] Chung[18] believes that the prognosis is good if treatment is begun within the first 2 days after the onset of symptoms. If the infection is untreated for several days, articular cartilage damage may lead to degenerative arthritis later in life.

Other disease processes affecting children may cause hip dysfunction. Hip girdle bleeding in hemophiliacs from muscular hemorrhage or hemarthrosis may cause a loss in hip ROM. Recurrent intraarticular bleeding may lead to chronic synovitis and degenerative joint disease.[21] Muscle weakness and contracture may develop. After bleeding has been stopped by bed rest and infusion of the coagulation factor, a gentle exercise program of ROM and strengthening may begin. At first, exercise should be limited to isometrics and active assistive exercises. Active resistive exercises should be added slowly after pain subsides.

Osteomyelitis, rheumatic fever, osteoid osteoma, and post-rubella immunization synovitis may also cause hip dysfunction in children.[18]

TRAUMATIC HIP PROBLEMS

Trauma to the developing hip joint may result in fractures, dislocations, ligamentous tears, muscular strains, and avascular necrosis.

Hip Fractures

In children, fractures are generally more common and tend to heal more rapidly than in adults. Torn ligaments and dislocations, on the other hand, are less common. Complications of fractures in children include growth disturbances, osteomyelitis, and refracture.[1]

Although rare, femoral neck fractures and injury to the proximal femoral epiphysis are serious owing to the risk of post-traumatic avascular necrosis. Considerable force, as from an automobile accident or a fall from a height, is required to cause a femoral neck fracture in a child.[6,7] Symptoms include hip pain, limited active motion, and resistance to passive motion. If the fracture is displaced, the limb may appear to be shortened and externally rotated.

Most fractures of the femoral neck require internal fixation, preceded by closed or open reduction if the fracture is displaced. Excessive hemorrhage is common.

Most femoral shaft fractures are treated nonsurgically.[7] Traction for a short time may be required to achieve good alignment before hip spica cast application.

Avulsion fractures, the result of forceful muscular contraction, may occur in the adolescent.[2] A contraction of the sartorius may avulse the anterior superior iliac spine, while the rectus femoris may avulse the anterior inferior spine. The gluteus medius and iliopsoas may avulse the greater and lesser trochanter, respectively. Point tenderness and pain at the avulsion site with active movement are common findings. Complete avulsion of the iliac spines may require internal fixation.[2] Avulsion of the greater trochanter may require stabilization in a hip spica cast.[6] Isometric exercise and gait training may be permitted after stabilization.

Traumatic Hip Dislocation

Traumatic posterior dislocation of the hip is rare in children but may occur from a force applied while the hip is flexed and adducted. The affected limb is held in flexion, adduction, and internal rotation with apparent shortening. Prompt reduction is essential to decrease the risk of avascular necrosis. A hip spica cast to maintain abduction and external rotation is usually required for approximately 8 weeks.[1]

A torn acetabular labrum may be a cause of hip pain.[22] A study by Dorrell and Catterall[23] considered it to be an acquired lesion in a mechanically weak dysplastic hip. This condition has been found in adolescents and young adults who had engaged in sports. The most common site for the tear was the posterior superior portion of the labrum. Symptoms may include pain on passive hip flexion and medial rotation. Diagnosis may be made by arthoscopy. Conservative treatment may include non-weightbearing for 6 to 12 weeks. Occasionally, partial resection of the labrum may be needed.

Snapping Hip

Snapping hip is a palpable, audible click noted with repetitive abduction and adduction. It is sometimes noted in infants (predominately female) and young women. This condition, which is painless, may be caused by the fascia lata sliding over the greater trochanter. Radiographs are normal, and no treatment is required.[4,18]

EVALUATION OF THE DEVELOPING HIP JOINT

Since detailed evaluation methods for hip joint dysfunction have been discussed in Chapter 2, only a few assessments specific to pediatrics will be discussed here.

Subjective data may be obtained from a variety of sources including verbal reports by the parent, teacher, or, depending on the child's age and development, the child. Additional information may be gained from medical records and direct observation of the child functioning in the environment. Pain may be assessed through vocal (e.g., crying), nonvocal (e.g., grimacing), physiologic (e.g., spasm), and avoidance (e.g., decreases play activity) behaviors.[24]

Objective data of hip dysfunction should include evaluation of the lower back, pelvis, and knee joint to ascertain whether these areas are functioning normally. When evaluating ROM in a child with spasticity, the measurements should reflect the child's functional range. Therefore, a realistic measurement would be the point at which resistance hinders passive movement, not the maximal range that may be obtained through resistive effort. Increased reliability of ROM may be achieved if measurements are taken at the same time in the treatment session. Measurement of hip abduction in the CP child with a windblown deformity can be difficult. A goniometeric system for measuring bilateral hip abduction in sitting has been developed to evaluate the hip joint and assess adaptive seating needs.[25] Specific strength tests may not be appropriate in some pediatric disorders; however, assessment of the child's movement patterns during function may be informative. The effect of the child's hip problem on the child's ability to move and function is key to any assessment.

Special tests for the pediatric population include those used to evaluate congenital hip dislocation. Ortolani's click, the Barlow test, and telescoping of the femur have been presented in Chapter 2.

TREATMENT CONSIDERATIONS

Nonsurgical treatment for the child with a hip disorder may include exercise programs, use of orthotics, casts, and adaptive devices, traction, medication, and bed rest.

A physical therapy program developed to meet the specific needs of a child with hip dysfunction (such as CHD, Legg-Calvé-Perthes disease, transient synovitis, and fracture) may include ROM, strengthening, pain control, and functional activities. A specific hip program may be only part of a total program for a child with multiple physical impairments (e.g., CP, JRA, myelomeningocele, and genetic disorders). Traction, casts, and orthosis are frequently used to treat CHD and Legg-Calvé-Perthes disease. A trochanteric girdle has been developed to prevent hip dislocation in standing for the child with severe acetabular dysplasia.[26] Use of crutches or other ambulatory aides and gait training may be appropriate for several hip disorders including Legg-Calvé-Perthes disease, slipped capital femoral epiphysis, transient synovitis, and hip fracture.

Adaptive seating systems that assist in maintenance of good postural alignment will promote hip stability. Proper seating is critical for any child who spends the majority of time in a wheelchair. A wheelchair with a solid seat and back such as the contoured positioning insert (Fig. 10-5) will provide more support than a standard sling seat wheelchair. A seating system that allows for hip, knee, and ankle positioning at 90° is desirable to ensure equal weight-bearing on the ischial tuberosities. A lumbar roll and lateral trunk supports may be needed to prevent pelvic obliquity. Abduction seating is recommended to maintain hip stability in a CP child prone to developing a windblown hip syndrome.[12]

Fig. 10-5. (**A**) Contoured positioning insert seating system. (**B**) Child with CP seated in contoured positioning insert system.

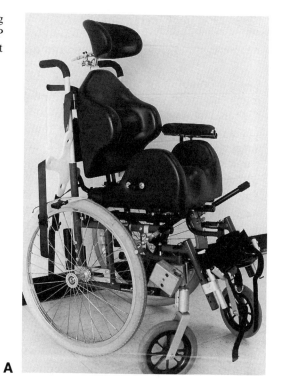

A

B

Surgical Procedures and Physical Therapy

Several of the pediatric hip problems discussed so far may require surgical intervention. Physical therapy pre- and postoperatively is often a vital part of the rehabilitation process.

Preoperatively, it is important that the child be prepared for an elective surgery both physically and psychologically.[27] Strength and endurance of the trunk and lower extremities should be maximized as much as possible before hip surgery. Parents or caregivers should be instructed in positioning techniques and handling skills (including cast management) before surgery. Special equipment needs such as a wheelchair, prone stander, or special underwear to accommodate a spica cast should be available before hospital discharge.

The child and family must also be prepared for the surgery psychologically. They need to understand the basic surgical procedure, the reason it is necessary, the estimated length of hospitalization, casting procedure (if applicable), and the expectation of pain. Showing the child books about going to the hospital may allay fears. Bringing some of the child's clothing, favorite foods, toys, and "lying down" activities will make the hospital stay more comfortable. Explain to the parents that the frequency of physical therapy often needs to be increased after surgery to maximize the benefits of surgery. If the child attends school, plans should be made for an immediate return after discharge to keep life as close to normal as possible.[27]

Adductor Tenotomy Transfer and the Anterior Obturator Neurectomy

This surgery is frequently indicated to lengthen a contracture or prevent (or slow) the tendency for hip dislocation. An adductor tenotomy involves selective cutting of some tendon fibers through an incision. (This may be done percutaneously when only 10° to 15° of abduction are needed.)[27] A transfer involves moving the adductor longus to the ischial tuberosity and a fascialotomy of the gracilis and adductor brevis. (Fig. 10-6). An anterior obturator neurectomy is sometimes done in combination with an adductor tenotomy. This nerve, which is dissected, arises from the second, third, and fourth lumbar nerves and innervates the adductor longus, brevis, and gracilis.[28] Matsuo et al.,[29] however, cautioned that with its dissection, the function of the adductor brevis is lost and hyperabduction and hip instability may result.

If the child is casted after the adductor surgery, the cast must maintain neutral hip extension and symmetry of both lower extremities in abduction.[27] This will help avoid hip flexion contracture or the windblown hip syndrome. The child should avoid sitting (1.5 hours per day maximum) to prevent hip flexor and quadriceps contracture and thoracic kyphosis. A prone or supine stander may be used for upright weightbearing. Walking in the cast, as the child is able, is usually permissible.[27] A hip spica cast may be required for about 3 weeks.[10]

If the child is not casted, gentle adductor stretching in functional activities

Fig. 10-6. Schematic drawing of position of transferred adductor muscles. (From Root,[10] with permission.)

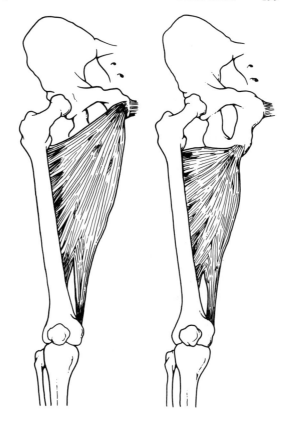

(e.g., reaching down between the legs while bench sitting) may be begun after discharge. Emphasis should be placed on active strengthening of the hip extensors and abductors in functional activities. If the noncasted child is nonambulatory, sitting activities should be limited to 1.5 hours per day for the first 2 weeks after surgery and use of a stander should be encouraged.[27]

Rectus Femoris and Tensor Fasciae Latae Tenotomy

Indications for a rectus femoris and tensor fasciae latae tenotomy include a 25° hip flexion contracture, increased quadriceps tone, poor sitting, exaggerated lordosis in walking, and a crouched gait or walking with a stiff knee and on the heels.[10] The aponeurosis of the tensor fasciae latae and tight fibers are transected, and the heads of the rectus femoris are detached (Fig. 10-7). According to Root,[10] the iliopsoas is not lengthened unless hip instability is present radiographically. This surgery may also be performed distally, by transferring the rectus femoris to the posterior medial or lateral tibia to better avoid knee instability.[27]

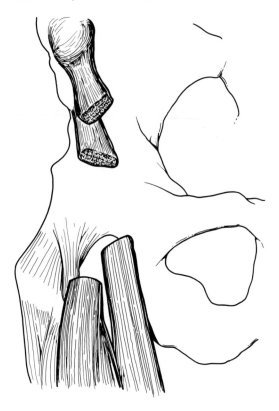

Fig. 10-7. Diagrammatic view of release of rectus femoris and sartorius. (From Root,[10] with permission.)

This procedure does not require casting, and ambulation and physical therapy may begin as soon as the patient is comfortable. Emphasis in treatment is placed on increasing knee flexion range within 15 days of the surgery, with ROM beginning after day 5 postoperatively.[27] Quadriceps strengthening should also be emphasized and may require 2 to 6 months before good active knee extension is achieved.

Hamstring Fascialotomy

Since tight hamstrings have a profound influence on the hip, pelvis, and sitting posture, their inclusion in this chapter seems appropriate. A functional range of 50° (tested by straight leg raising, maintaining 0° knee extension) is needed for a normal stride length in gait.[27] Usually the medial hamstrings are more involved and may contribute to hip internal rotation as well. This surgical procedure usually involves incision into the gracilis and some of the semitendinosus fibers. Only the aponeurosis of the semimembranosus is incised. It is recommended that this procedure be performed early (around 3 years of age) before biomechanical changes occur.[27] It frequently needs to be repeated later as the child grows.

Occasionally the child is placed in a cylinder cast for 1 or 2 weeks. If not casted, care must be taken to maintain knee extension during healing. Standing with or without casts should be encouraged immediately after surgery. Gait training, trunk activities, and ball gymnastics are recommended. The child should avoid toe touching during healing. To prevent hip flexion and quadriceps contractures, quadriceps strengthening in the cast and prolonged sitting (over 1.5 hours per day) should be avoided.[27]

Varus Femoral Rotation Osteotomy

Varus femoral rotation osteotomy is a complex surgical procedure that may be indicated to correct hip dislocation, excessive femoral anteversion, and increase angle of inclination (coxa valga).[8] The procedure involves removing a wedge of bone from the medial side of the femur at the level of the lesser trochanter and stabilizing the bone in its new position with a compression plate. (Fig. 10-8). Stabilization is similar to the procedure used in repairing a

Fig. 10-8. Schematic view of varus rotation osteotomy redirecting the femoral head centrally into the acetabulum. (From Root,[10] with permission.)

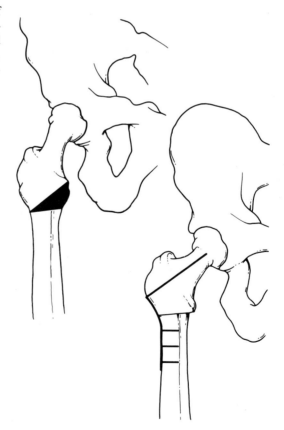

subtrochanteric fracture in the elderly. Postoperative problems may include limb shortening and compensatory external tibial torsion.

A hip spica cast with hip extension at 0° may be required for about 3 weeks.[10] Treatment during the casted period may include active and passive back extension and upper extremity exercise. Some orthopaedists may permit standing and gait activities while in the cast. Sitting should be avoided.

After cast removal, the child may resume sitting activities and active ROM may be initiated. Weightbearing may be gradually increased. At 6 weeks, if the osteotomy is well healed, ambulation and nonrestricted activities may begin.[10] The child is usually very weak after this procedure and may lose some sitting ability. Knee flexion is usually painful. Active hip extension, abduction, external rotation, and flexion beyond 90° (within 2 weeks of cast removal) should be encouraged. Functional activities like bench sitting with trunk movement and transitional movements should be emphasized. Prone positioning to maintain hip extension should be stressed at home for 80 percent of the day after cast removal.[27] Adduction past neutral and internal rotation should be avoided to prevent stress on the compression plate.

Occasionally a child may not be casted for this procedure. In that case, the child must maintain non-weightbearing (no standing or walking) for 3 weeks after surgery.[27]

Selective Dorsal Rhizotomy

This relatively new neurosurgical procedure is designed to decrease the influence of spasticity in the lower extremities in children with CP. Since many hip problems in CP are related to hypertonicity and muscle imbalance, the inclusion of this procedure seems appropriate in discussing hip problems.

Selective dorsal rhizotomy involves selective cutting of the dorsal (sensory) rootlets in the lumbar spine that are determined to cause spasticity. This determination is made from electomyographic responses from stimulated rootlets. Normal rootlets are left intact. Candidates for surgery include children over 2 years of age with spastic diplegia, hemiplegia, or quadriplegia in which spasticity limits their functional abilities.[30] The parents must be committed to an intense program of physical therapy at least two to four times a week for 1 year after the surgery. Children with athetosis, dystonia, or scoliosis or those who have had several orthopaedic surgeries are not considered good candidates.[30] Complications may include paralysis, wound infection, and meningitis.

A preoperative physical therapy evaluation should include developmental history, developmental function, quality of gait, ROM, and the influence of spasticity on functional abilities.

Postoperatively, the child is on strict bed rest for 5 days. Mat activities including rolling, bridging, prone propping, and gentle stretching may begin on day 6. Lower extremity weightbearing can often begin on day 10. Restrictions include vigorous hamstring stretching and passive trunk movements into the extremes of range.[30]

Physical therapy goals include improving postural alignment and balance, increasing lower extremity ROM and strength, developing isolated lower extremity movements, and improving function in gait, transitions, and newly acquired skills.

SUMMARY

Hip problems in children differ from those in the adult owing to the immaturity of their musculoskeletal system. Pediatric hip problems may be classified into four areas: congenital, developmental, disease processes, and traumatic occurrences. Specific hip problems in each category, evaluation procedures, and treatment methods, both surgical and nonsurgical, were discussed. Emphasis was placed on early intervention to prevent deformity and maximize function.

REFERENCES

1. Salter R: Textbook of Disorders and Injuries of the Musculoskeletal System. 2nd Ed. Williams & Wilkins, Baltimore, 1983
2. Saudek C: The hip. p. 365. In Gould JA, Davies GJ (eds): Orthopaedic and Sports Physical Therapy. CV Mosby, St. Louis, 1985
3. LeVeau B, Bernhardt D: Developmental biomechanics. Phys Ther 64:1874, 1984
4. Ramey R, Brashear HR: Shand's Handbook of Orthopaedic Surgery. 8th Ed. CV Mosby, St. Louis, 1971
5. Hoppenfield S: Physical Examination of the Spine and Extremities. Appleton-Century-Crofts, Norwalk, CT, 1976
6. Tachdjian M: Pediatric Orthopedics. WB Saunders, Philadelphia, 1972
7. Scoles P: Pediatric Orthopedics in Clinical Practice. 2nd Ed. Year Book Medical Publishers, Chicago, 1988
8. Hensinger RN: Congenital dislocation of the hip—treatment in infancy to walking age. Orthop Clin North Am 18:597, 1987
9. Jones E, Knapp D: Assessment and management of the lower extremity in cerebral palsy. Orthop Clin North Am 18:725, 1987
10. Root L: Treatment of hip problems in cerebral palsy. Instr Course Lect 36:237, 1987
11. Cooperman D, Bartucci E, Dietrick E, et al: Hip dislocation in spastic cerebral palsy—long term consequences. J Pediatr Orthop 7:268, 1987
12. Letts M, Shapiro L, Molder K, et al: The windblown hip syndrome in total body C.P. J Pediatr Orthop 4:55, 1984
13. Carroll N: Assessment and management of the lower extremity in myelodysplasia. Orthop Clin North Am 18:709, 1987
14. Sherk H, Melchienne J, Smith R: The natural history of hip dislocation in ambulatory myelomenigocele. Z Kinderchir 422:48, 1987
15. Weisl H, Fairchough J, Jones D: Stabilization of the hip in myelomeningocele: Comparison of posterior iliopsoas transfer and varus rotation osteotomy. J Bone Joint Surg 70:29, 1988
16. Staheli L, Chew D, Elliott J, et al: Management of hip dislocations in children with arthrogryposis. J Pediatr Orthop 7:681, 1987

17. Harris S, Tada W: Genetic Disorders in Children. p. 184. In Umphred D (ed): Neurological Rehabilitation. CV Mosby, St. Louis, 1985
18. Chung S: Diseases of the developing hip joint. Pediatr Clin North Am 33:1457, 1986
19. Rodnan G, Schumacher H, Zvaifler N: Juvenile rheumatoid arthritis. p. 97. In Rodnan G, Schumacher H (eds): Primer on the Rheumatic Diseases. 8th Ed. Arthritis Foundation, Atlanta, 1983
20. Blane C, Ragsdale C, Hensinger R: Late effects of JRA on the hip. J Pediatr Orthop 7:677, 1987
21. Goodman S, Gamble J, Dilley M: Hip motion changes in hemophilia. J Pediatr Orthop 7:664, 1987
22. Ikeda T, Awaya G, Suzuki, S, et al: Torn acetabular labrum in young patients. J Bone Joint Surg 70:12, 1988
23. Dorrell J, Catterall A: The torn acetabular labrum. J Bone Joint Surg 68B:400, 1986
24. Lavigre J, Schulein M, Hannan J, et al: Pain and the pediatric patient: Psychological aspects. p. 267. In Echternach JL (ed): Pain. Churchill Livingstone, New York, 1987
25. Nwaobi OM: Goniometer system for measuring bilateral hip abduction in children with C.P.: Suggestion from the field. Phys Ther 67:953, 1987
26. Ruys E: Trochanteric girdle to prevent hip dislocation in standing: Suggestion from the field. Phys Ther 68:226, 1988
27. McGee M: Selected aspects of orthopedic surgery management for the person with cerebral palsy. Instr Course Lect 1988
28. Goss CM: Gray's Anatomy. 29th Ed. p. 987. Lea & Febiger, Philadelphia, 1975
29. Matsuo T, Tada S, Hajime T: Insufficiency of the hip adductor after anterior obturator neurectomy in 42 children with C.P. J Pediatr Orthop 6:686, 1986
30. Park TS, Payne MO, Wilson J, et al: Selective Dorsal Rhizotomy: A Neurosurgical Approach in Spasticity in Cerebral Palsy Children—A Guidebook for Parents. University of Virginia, Charlottesville, 1988

11 | Geriatric Hip Problems

John L. Echternach, Jr.

As members of the health care community, physical therapists must stay abreast of current trends. One trend that will have a significant impact on virtually all aspects of health care, including physical therapy, is the projected increase in the elderly population. Lewis[1] noted that in the late 1800s only 3 percent of the U.S. population was 65 years of age, by 1985 11 percent were 65 or over, and by the year 2020 30 percent will be 65 or older. Jette[2] in 1986 reported that the population of elderly 85 or over had increased by 140 percent between 1960 and 1980. Kart et al.[3] noted that this elderly population will be predominantly female, with a ratio of 72 males/100 females.

Obviously physical therapists can expect to see a steady increase in elderly patients seeking care. Lewis[1] observed that the elderly are significant consumers of all forms of health care; people over 65 visit the doctor 43 percent more often than those under 65.

This chapter explores one aspect of geriatrics—common hip problems in the elderly. It covers two specific areas: first, typical hip joint degenerative changes with age, and second, hip problems in the aging population. Within each area the etiology, medical and surgical treatment, and physical therapy intervention are discussed. Also, the effects of recent changes in the health care system on the delivery of care for these patients is discussed briefly.

DEGENERATIVE JOINT DISEASE

Degenerative joint disease (DJD), or osteoarthritis, can be defined as a local and progressive deterioration of articular cartilage and subchondral bone and inflammation of the synovium. DJD is most common in weightbearing joints. It can also be divided into two categories: primary and secondary. Primary DJD refers to changes caused by the normal aging process, while secondary DJD refers to a related or prior disease or injury of a joint. Examples could include congenital dislocation, hip fracture, and traumatic dislocation.

Typical complaints or symptoms of osteoarthritis include joint pain, stiffness, and swelling, which can limit active motion. Crepitation (palpable and sometimes audible crackling with joint motion) is often present.[4] Radiographic evidence of joint degeneration is considered the most reliable clinical sign of DJD.[4,5] Several sources state that radiographic evidence of DJD in the extremities is seen almost universally in the population aged 65 and over.[4,5] However, Masi and Medsger[5] found that only about 30 percent of individuals with radiographic evidence of DJD at that site complain of pain. This finding correlates well with that of Kart et al.,[3] who stated that by age 60, 25 percent of women and 15 percent of men have symptoms of DJD. Masi and Medsger[5] and Saudek[6] noted an increased incidence of DJD in older women.

Etiology

In a review of the literature three primary theories regarding the etiology of DJD are encountered: (1) altered biomechanics, (2) excessive use or wear and tear, and (3) prolonged immobilization or disuse.[6–8]

Altered biomechanics of the hip joint and resulting DJD would be considered an example of secondary DJD. Predisposing factors could include Legg-Calvé-Perthes disease, which results in alteration of the shape of the femoral head. Cooperman et al.[7] reported that long-term prognosis was related to shape of the femoral head at skeletal maturity. Patients with a more rounded femoral head at maturity had normal hip function at long-term follow up. Patients whose femoral head was more square or flattened at skeletal maturity had increased loss of function at long-term follow up. Another predisposing factor could be a vascular necrosis of the head of the femur following hip fracture.[6] As a consequence of the necrosis, the shape of the femoral head becomes flattened and irregularly shaped.

The opposing theories of wear and tear and disuse as causes of DJD both hinge on the response of articular cartilage to compression forces. Leveau and Bernhard[8] noted that high compression forces cause cartilage degeneration while an absence of compression leads to atrophy. These observations led to the conclusion that regular or "normal" use of a joint provides for adequate cartilage maintenance while regular and excessive compression or a total lack of compression disrupt cartilage maintenance and lead to degeneration. Once degeneration has begun, excessive forces tend to accelerate the degenerative process.

Several studies have explored the wear and tear/overuse theory of DJD. Pinals[9] and Moskowitz[10] reported on several studies correlating DJD and repetitive occupational trauma, primarily in hands and upper extremities. These reviews reported on increased DJD in ankles of soccer players and in the knees of miners. However, it was found that competitive running did not predispose athletes to DJD of the hip. Intuitively some of the correlations between repetitive work trauma and DJD make sense, but more study is needed to define what constitutes an excessive load for a particular joint. Unfortunately no studies correlated the effect of prolonged immobilization to developing DJD.

Typical DJD Changes in the Hip

Degenerative changes in the hip joint tend to follow a typical progression. Initially the articular cartilage begins to lose proteoglycan from its matrix. This causes a general softening of the cartilage and decreases its resilience and ability to respond to stress. Eventually this leads to increased friction of the collagen fibers, causing them to shred and progressing to fissures and splits in the cartilage. Ultimately cartilage wears away to subchondral bone, especially in the upper quadrant of the femoral head, which is the area of greatest contact on weightbearing.

As subchondral bone is exposed it tends to hypertrophy, becoming polished and denser. In the peripheral joint areas, cartilage tends to hypertrophy and ossify, forming osteophytes or bony spurs and lipping at the joint margins. All of the above changes tend to alter the distribution of weightbearing forces, eventually causing the femoral head and acetabulum to become flattened. A decrease in jointspace is also seen radiographically. Synovitis can also develop owing to increased strain on the joint capsule and as an inflammatory reaction to cartilage breakdown.

The most common complaint with DJD of the hip is pain upon weightbearing. Pain can be localized to the hip region or radiate into the thigh and knee. Patients often report stiffness and decreased active hip motion. The affected hip is often held in a position of flexion, adduction, and external rotation because of fibrotic changes in the joint capsule. In some cases the affected leg may be shortened, leading to leg-length discrepancy and possibly resulting in low back pain.

Treatment

Treatment for hip DJD is multifaceted. Use of an assistive device for ambulation should be discussed with the patient. This could help decrease weightbearing forces on the affected hip and allow the patient to remain ambulatory with less discomfort. The patient should be instructed in exercises to strengthen all muscle groups about the hip. The exercises should be monitored initially with the goal of the patient's performing them daily in the home. Joint mobilization can be effective in reducing joint capsule tightness and increasing specific motions. Heat treatment before exercise can help to decrease stiffness and pain, making exercise more comfortable. If a patient has a significant leg length discrepancy, a shoe lift will often help decrease excessive weightbearing forces on the hips and decrease pain. Patients can often benefit from general conditioning exercises, such as walking or swimming, for aerobic as well as range of motion (ROM) benefits.

It is especially important to counsel the patient regarding the proper balance between rest and exercise. If patients perceive increased pain over $\frac{1}{2}$ hour postexercise they have probably exceeded their tolerance. It is important for the therapist to monitor patients' responses to exercise and help them progress their exercise programs to the appropriate level. Spreading activity over the entire day with periodic brief rest periods can also help. Patients should realize that exercise will not cure their arthritis. However, a regular exercise program can be instrumental in maintaining joint mobility and fitness and preventing disabling joint contractures and debilitation.

Drug therapy is also an important aspect of managing DJD.[11] Analgesic drugs such as aspirin (acetylsalicylic acid) and acetaminophen help to decrease pain. Nonsteroidal anti-inflammatory drugs help to control synovial inflammation. Commonly prescribed anti-inflammatory drugs include indomethacin, ibuprofen, fenoprofen, and naprosyntolectin. Intra-articular injection of steroids is used occasionally to treat joint pain in DJD. Pain relief varies, lasting a few days to several months. Some investigators have noted that injections to the hip were least effective when compared with other joints.[11]

Total Hip Replacement

In advanced cases of hip DJD with structural damage to the joint, total hip replacement has become a common procedure. Rodnan and Schumacher[4] suggest that a conservative course of physical therapy (as outlined previously) and drugs be tried to maintain function at acceptable levels. If this is not successful then surgery may be considered. Information about total hip replacements is discussed in Chapter 5. The role of the physical therapist in the care of the patient with a total hip replacement is fully discussed in Chapter 6. A brief review with emphasis on the older patient is offered here.

A preoperative visit by the physical therapist is helpful to discuss postoperative exercises and the ambulation program and to review precautions such as no hip flexion greater than 90°, no adduction past midline, and no excessive internal or external rotation following surgery. The patient can begin a program of isometrics and active motion exercises as soon after surgery as practical. It is important to communicate with the surgeon regarding any specific motion and weightbearing restrictions that apply to a particular patient. Patients will begin ambulation with a walker following surgery. Precautions on hip motion should be reviewed postoperatively and the patients instructed in the proper techniques of rolling in bed, coming to sitting and standing, and performing daily activities while adhering to these precautions.

The physical therapist plays an important role in working with elderly patients who have hip DJD. The therapist works closely with the patient to design an exercise program to maintain hip strength and mobility. The therapist also assists in evaluating and providing the appropriate assistive devices for ambulation.

HIP FRACTURES IN THE ELDERLY

Hip fracture (proximal femur fracture) is a significant cause of death and disability among the elderly. Wallace[12] noted a steady increase in hip fracture incidence from 8 out of 1000 to 16 out of 1000 between 1971 and 1981. Hielema[13] and Lewinnek et al.[14] reported increased incidence of hip fracture in females, especially in the 75 years and over age group. Bollet[15] found that the hip fracture rate for whites was twice that of blacks. Therefore it seems that the typical hip fracture patient would be a white female 75 years or older. As the number of elderly increase in the general population, physical therapists can expect to deal with a steady and significant increase in hip fracture patients.

Predispositions and Causes of Hip Fracture

The most common cause of hip fracture in the elderly is accidental falls. Chipman and Saran[16] and Rodstein[17] reported that falls constitute the single largest cause of accidental death in the elderly. Many of these falls would be considered trivial in a younger person, but the elderly individual often is predisposed to a serious injury from falling by one or more factors including osteoporosis, decrease in visual acuity, circulatory disorders, and musculoskeletal system changes.[17]

Osteoporosis is a generalized decrease in bone mass often seen in the elderly, especially women.[18] Factors in osteoporosis include increased calcium resorption, decreased calcium deposition, lack of calcium in diet, and inactivity. Block[19] et al. reviewed the literature on exercise and osteoporosis: one study found a significant correlation between aerobic capacity and bone mass in the lumbo-sacral spine and the femoral neck. Another found that in a group of 1,200 women, the 124 most active women had a significant increase in bone mass at all ages compared with the other women in the study. Block et al.[19] surmised that regular exercise may reduce the number of falls and decrease serious injury in falls. Riis et al.[20] found estrogen treatment prevented bone loss in postmenopausal women while calcium supply only slowed it. They also noted that combining low dose estrogen and calcium prevented bone loss in postmenopausal women. Low dose estrogen was felt to be more effective in decreasing secondary gynecologic effects.

Also of importance are the trabecular patterns in the bone of the femoral head and neck. Kessler and Hertling[21] noted an area of inherent weakness in the femoral neck region (Fig. 11-1). When combined with osteoporosis, this can predispose this region to a fracture.

Elderly persons often show changes in their visual systems that could lead to a fall. These include a loss of peripheral vision, decreased visual acuity, and a general need for increased illumination.[22] These changes are often very gradual and the individual may not be consciously aware of visual losses. Preventive measures could include regular vision checks by a physician to alert patients of

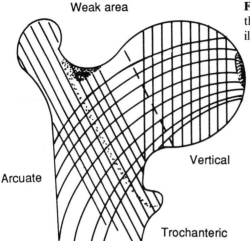

Weak area

Arcuate

Vertical

Trochanteric

Fig. 11-1. The trabecular patterns of the bone of the femoral head and neck, illustrating the weak area.

changes and their implications. Increasing lighting in and around the home could be helpful, especially in hallways and around steps and walks.

Atherosclerosis and orthostatic hypotension are circulatory disorders that can cause dizzy spells in the elderly. Atherosclerosis of the carotid and vertebral arteries may be associated with dizzy spells in specific head positions, especially extending the head back (vertebral artery) or rotating the head to the left or right (carotids). The best way to deal with this problem is to identify it and educate the patient to avoid these head positions. In the elderly, the blood pressure regulatory mechanism works more slowly and may cause orthostatic hypotension.[23] Consequently standing quickly from a sitting or lying position may cause a temporary disruption in blood flow to the brain. Older persons have to train themselves to change position more slowly to allow the body's blood pressure regulators time to work.

General musculoskeletal system changes with age include diminished proprioception, decreased coordination of movement, and slowing of reflexes. These changes are usually attributed to decreased blood supply to brain, spinal cord, and peripheral nerves.[24–26] These changes together often produce a shuffling gait in which the feet barely lift off the floor. This places the individual at risk for tripping over the smallest obstacle. Floor space in the home should be as clear as possible to prevent this from occurring. Thresholds, throw rugs, extension cords, and the like should be removed if possible.

Fracture Type and Therapy

Naylor[26] described three main types of hip fracture: subcapital, transcervical, and intertrochanteric (Fig. 11-2). Subcapital and transcervical fractures occur at the base of the femoral head and are contained within the joint capsule.

Fig. 11-2. The sites of the three main types of hip fracture: Subcapital, trans-cervical, and intertrochanteric.

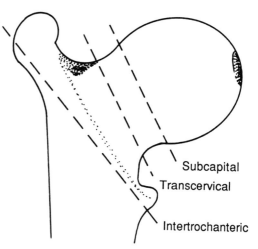

Subcapital

Transcervical

Intertrochanteric

These fractures frequently present a problem of significant change in articular cartilage or nonunion owing to disruption of blood supply to the femoral head. Because of these complications, surgeons may prefer prosthetic replacement of the femoral head and neck (hemi-arthroplasty) over internal fixation.[27] This involves removing the bony head and neck of the femur above the greater trochanter and cementing a prosthesis in the femoral canal. An advantage of the hemi-arthroplasty is greatly reduced recovery time. A long wait for bony union is unnecessary, so patients can generally begin ambulation sooner, tolerate increased weightbearing, and experience less pain with activity.

Intertrochanteric fractures are located outside the joint capsule. As this area is well supplied with blood vessels, fracture union is seldom a problem. Intertrochanter fractures are generally treated surgically by open reduction and internal fixation. This involves a posterolateral incision on the hip to expose the joint.[26] The fracture is aligned visually and radiographically. Then a nail or screw is inserted to hold the fracture fragments in alignment. The nail or screw is often supplemented by a plate attached to the nail/screw head and to the femoral shaft.[26]

While internal fixation allows the patient to begin ambulation within a week, often the weightbearing on the affected limb must be restricted for extended periods to allow bony union to occur. Pain with ambulation or active motion can also be a factor in limiting early mobility or restricting function.[26] Some orthopaedic surgeons delay weightbearing in an effort to decrease avascular necrosis while others feel that early weightbearing can enhance the patient's rehabilitation potential.[28,29]

An occasional late (6 to 12 months) complication of hip fracture repaired by open reduction and internal fixation is trochanteric bursitis. This results from the nail or screw projecting from the bone into the soft tissues around the greater trochanter. The resulting pain on weightbearing on the affected limb can necessitate removal of the nail or screw used for fixation.

Rehabilitation

The primary objectives of a rehabilitation program are to achieve painless stability, adequate ROM, and maximum function in the affected limb.[27,30-32] Ideally, the rehabilitation program should start before surgery. At this time the physician or therapist should explain the operation, the postoperative exercise program and, in general terms, what outcome the patient can expect. Also at this time it is important to explain postoperative movements to be avoided, such as bending the hip beyond 90° and crossing the ankles or knees.

Postoperative exercise is aimed at strengthening the hip flexors, extensors, abductors, and adductors of the affected leg. This is combined with work on ambulation skills and transfer technique to enable the patient to perform activities of daily living. Exercise programs are also carried out to maintain strength and range of motion in the unaffected leg. The upper extremities are also exercised to prepare for the demands of using a walker or crutches.

Postoperative exercises on a day-by-day basis would be as follows:

Days 1 through 3. The patient is primarily in bed following a program of isometric setting exercise of the quadriceps, gluteal, and hamstring muscle groups. The patient is also encouraged to put the feet and ankles through active range of motion to encourage circulation. The patient should perform these exercises at least once or twice daily with a therapist and be encouraged to perform them alone as often as tolerated.

Days 3 through 5. The patient is started on a program of active assistive flexion, extension, abduction, and adduction of the affected limb. Strength of the hip abductors is especially important to emphasize in an exercise program, more so than other muscle groups. Barnes and Donovan[33] found a significant correlation between hip abductor strength and the ability to ambulate independently. The therapist should perform these exercises with the patient at least once daily and encourage the patient to perform them alone as tolerated. Providing the patient with slings or a sliding board to assist with the exercises will aid in performing them in bed. At this point the patient is encouraged to spend part of the day sitting.

One week after surgery. The patient can usually begin training in ambulation and transfers. Ambulation is most frequently partial weightbearing on the affected limb as determined in consultation with the surgeon. Ambulation training is usually begun with a walker since the patient will be on limited weightbearing to no weightbearing. As patients progress to full weightbearing on the affected limb, they should be evaluated for progressing to other assistive devices such as crutches. The patient's safety, stability, and need for independence must all be considered. If stability is at all in question, the patient should probably remain on a walker. Barnes and Donovan[33] reported that in a group of 67 hip fracture patients followed through to final discharge, only 15 progressed to using a cane.

Early discharge from the hospital is becoming more commonplace. Consequently many patients will benefit from continuing treatment, possibly in a rehabilitation facility, in the home, or as outpatients. Early discharge becomes an important issue for the physical therapist when designing a treatment program for the hip fracture patient; what are reasonable goals/outcomes to expect and what variables can have useful predictive value?

A few studies have examined this question. Cedar et al.[34] found that patients with no medical complications and the ability to ambulate 2 weeks after surgery were highly correlated with return to independent living. Barnes and Donovan[33] reported that increased age (85 or above), lower extremity contracture, weak hip abductors, and a history of stroke were all associated with dependence in ambulation. These studies highlight several important points. First, the importance of early mobilization to prevent contractures and general debilitation. It is common knowledge that the elderly patient is much more prone to rapid loss of muscle strength and decreased ROM when confined to bed. Second, even in the ambulatory patient, it is important to maintain ROM and strengthen the affected limb. If rapid fatigue is a problem, then resistive exercise needs to focus most on the hip abductors. The abductors, important in stabilizing the pelvis when ambulating, are significantly weakened as a result of surgery. When evaluating a hip fracture patient, careful documentation of ROM and strength (especially of the affected lower extremity) and thorough chart review should provide baseline data. Regular reassessment of the patient's response to treatment should allow the therapist to be accurate and realistic in setting goals and outcomes.

Fitzgerald et al.[35] documented important trends in the care of elderly hip fracture patients, especially in regard to diagnostic related groups (DRG) and early hospital discharge. They found that length of hospital stay had decreased from 21 days before DRG to 12 days after implementation of DRG. They also noted that 30 percent fewer patients were ambulatory at time of hospital discharge and there was a 60 percent increase in patients placed in nursing homes. Most significant was their finding of a 200 percent increase in long-term nursing home residence after hospital discharge. Most patients in nursing homes at 1 year follow-up required skilled care, indicating they had not regained strength and endurance needed for independent living.[35] What does this all mean? First, that the setting for care of the elderly hip fracture patient is shifting from the hospital to outside settings, such as nursing homes, home health, and outpatient care. Second, Fitzgerald et al.[35] suggest that informal rehabilitation by hospital nursing staff and family may play a part. This may be a crucial point. Once the therapist has instructed staff and family on how to assist a patient with activities of daily living and ambulation, they are responsible for implementing these activities as part of the patient's schedule. This may not be possible in the nursing home environment.

SUMMARY

The role of the physical therapist in the management and care of the elderly patient with hip problems can be expected to increase in the future. The major reasons for this are the increasing numbers of elderly members of our society who will require care and the increasing responsibilities of the physical therapist in providing care for the musculoskeletal problems associated with aging.

REFERENCES

1. Lewis C (Ed.): Aging, The Health Care Challenge. F.A. Davis Co., Philadelphia, 1985
2. Jette A: Functional disability and rehabilitation of the aged. Top Geriatr Rehabil 1:1, 1986
3. Kart C, Metress E, Metress J: Aging and Health, Biologic and Social Perspectives. Addison-Wesley Publishing, Reading, MA, 1978
4. Rodnan G, Schumacher R: Primer on the Rheumatic Disease. Arthritis Foundation, Atlanta, 1983
5. Masi A, Medsger T: Epidemiology of rheumatic diseases. In McCarty D (Ed.): Arthritis and Allied Conditions. Lea & Febiger, Philadelphia, 1979
6. Saudek C: The hip. p. 365. In Gould JA, Davies GJ (eds.): Orthopedic and Sports Physical Therapy. CV Mosby, St. Louis, 1985
7. Cooperman D, Emery H, Keller C: Factors relating to hip joint arthritis following three childhood diseases, juvenile rheumatoid arthritis, perthes disease and post reduction avascular necrosis in congenital hip dislocation. J Pediatr Orthop 6:706, 1986
8. Leveau B, Bernhard D: Developmental biomechanics, effect of forces on the growth, development and maintenance of the human body. Phys Ther 64:1874, 1984
9. Pinals R: Traumatic arthritis and allied conditions. In McCarty D (Ed.): Arthritis and Allied Conditions. Lea & Febiger, Philadelphia, 1979
10. Moskowitz R: Clinical and laboratory findings in osteoarthritis. In McCarty D (Ed.): Arthritis and Allied Conditions. Lea & Febiger, Philadelphia, 1979
11. Moskowitz R: Treatment of osteoarthritis. In McCarty D (Ed.): Arthritis and Allied Conditions. Lea & Febiger, Philadelphia, 1979
12. Wallace W: The increasing incidence of fracture of the proximal femur: An orthopedic epidemic. Lancet 1:1413, 1983
13. Hielema F: Epidemiology of hip fracture, a review for physical therapists. Phys Ther 9:1221, 1979
14. Lewinnek G, Kelsey J, White A, Kreiger N: The significance and a comparative analysis of the epidemiology of hip fracture. Clin Orthop 152, 1980
15. Bollet S: Epidemiology of osteoporosis. Arch Intern Med 116:191, 1965
16. Chipman C, Saran D: What does it mean when a patient falls? Pinpointing the cause. Geriatrics 36:83, 1981
17. Rodstein M: Accidents among the aged. In Reichel W (Ed.): Clinical Aspects of Aging. Williams & Wilkins, Baltimore, 1978
18. Barzel V: Common metabolic disorders of the skeleton in aging. In Reichel W (Ed.): Clinical Aspects of Aging. Williams & Wilkins, Baltimore, 1978
19. Block J, Smith R, Black D, Genant H: Does exercise prevent osteoporosis? JAMA 257 (22):345, 1987
20. Riis B, Thomsen K, Christiansen C: Does calcium supplementation prevent post menopausal bone loss? N Engl J Med 316 (7):360, 1987
21. Kessler R, Hertling D: Management of Common Musculoskeletal Disorders. Harper & Row, New York, 1983

22. Kaspar R: Eye Problems of the Aged. In Reichel W (Ed.): Clinical Aspects of Aging. Williams & Wilkins, Baltimore, 1978

23. Exton-Smith A: Disorders of the Autonomic Nervous System. In Castro F (Ed.): Neurological Disorders in the Elderly. Wright & Sons, Bristol, 1982

24. Isaacs B: Disorders of balance. In Castro F (Ed.): Neurological Disorders in the Elderly. Wright & Sons, Bristol, 1982

25. Grob D: Common disorders of muscle in the aged. In Reichel W (Ed.): Clinical Aspects of Aging. Williams & Wilkins, Baltimore, 1978

26. Naylor A: Fractures and Orthopedic Surgery for Physiotherapists. Williams & Wilkins, Baltimore, 1968

27. Watkins A: Management of hip disabilities. Arch Phys Med Rehab 35:247, 1954

28. Blount J: Don't throw away the cane. J Bone Joint Surg 38A:695, 1956

29. Clawson D, Welcher P: Fractures and dislocations of the hip. In Rockwood C and Green D (Ed.): Fractures. Vol. 2. JB Lippincott, Philadelphia, 1975

30. Gucker T: Exercise in orthopedics. In Light J (Ed.): Therapeutic Exercise. Williams & Wilkins, Baltimore, 1965

31. Rusk H: Rehabilitation Medicine. CV Mosby, St. Louis, 1977

32. Taniguchi S: Physical therapy program for a patient with an Austin Moore prosthesis. Phys Ther 41:118, 1959

33. Barnes B, Donovan K: Physical therapy discharge outcomes after hip fracture. Top Geriatr Rehabil 2(4):45, 1987

34. Cedar L, Thorgren KG, Wallden B: Prognostic indicators and early home rehabilitation in elderly patients with hip fractures. Clin Orthop 152:173, 1980

35. Fitzgerald J, Moore P, Dittus R: The care of elderly patients with hip fracture, changes since implementation of the prospective payment system. N Engl J Med 319:1392, 1988

Index

Page numbers followed by *f* designate figures and those followed by *t* designate tables.